PRAISE FOR *STAGE OF FOOLS*

"Sean Pauzauskie is from that great tradition of doctors who also excel in literature. As with Walker Percy, another example, we get in Pauzauskie's *Stage of Fools* the tragicomedies of the flesh as well as the acutely sketched-out questions about the mind and the soul. Sean Pauzauskie is a very promising novelist, with a big heart and unique angle, as shown in this uniquely rewarding new work."

—Rick Moody, author of *The Ice Storm*

"*Stage of Fools* offers an innovative, compelling appropriation and repurposing of Shakespeare's *King Lear*. But the principal character lies comatose in a San Francisco hospital, able to hear, think, and feel. Recollection and disintegration drive a bold family narrative toward a riveting conclusion and epiphany. Pauzauskie, by creating multi-faceted characters, skillfully refashions the story of an old king into a modern-day enriched parable of hope, suffering, and loss."

—David Bergeron, author of *The Duke of Lennox*

"Sean Pauzauskie's *Stage of Fools* is not just a medical thriller and murder mystery, it's also an inventive and provocative mediation on the beauty of human consciousness. Narrated by the unforgettable Steve Levinson, this novel is compelling, smart, and wildly entertaining."

—Lewis Robinson, author of *Waterdogs*

"A wild ride into the far reaches of inner space, where the chaos of the mind competes with the messes of the world, all unfolding under the deft hand of Pauzauskie and his literary, intellectual, medical, and historical expertise. As madness and reason collide, the novel reverberates with the lament of King Lear—"O, let me not be mad, not mad, sweet heaven!"—as it explores the boundaries of consciousness and sanity in an unraveling world. Fasten your seatbelts!"

—Brett Shapiro, author of *L'Intruso*

STAGE OF FOOLS

A NOVEL

SEAN PAUZAUSKIE

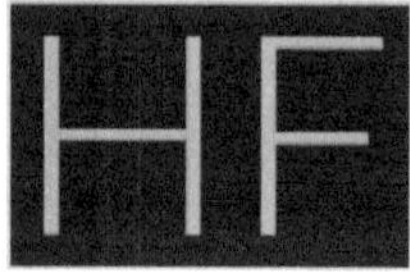

HIGH FREQUENCY PRESS

Published by High Frequency Press
www.highfrequencypress.com

Postal mail may be sent to:
High Frequency Press
PO Box 472
Brunswick, ME 04011

ISBN: 978-1-962931-31-1
LCCN: 2025905204

Printed in the United States of America

For Dad, and Pan

"When we are born, we cry that we are come to this great stage of fools."

—William Shakespeare
King Lear, Act IV, scene VI

STAGE OF FOOLS

DRAMATIS PERSONÆ

THOMAS MARINER, a fine young man.
STEVEN LEVINSON, a business magnate.
CARMELIA, wife to Levinson.
DANNY, son to Levinson.

DR. JANE EUGENE, a neurologist.
HERMAN, father to Levinson.
BREINA, mother to Levinson.
DMITRI BUGAEV, a business partner to Herman.
ETHAN HELMS, a childhood friend to Levinson.
ELIE MONROE, beloved of Danny, and Thomas.

Fool.

VLADIMIR, son to Bugaev.
NATALYA, daughter to Bugaev.
KIRA, daughter to Natalya.

CAMILLE LE, beloved of Levinson.
HAO LE, guardian to Camille.

FERRIS BUNDY, a rogue.
HARRY FRANK, a bear hunting guide.
RICH DAWSON, a tourist, and psychologist.
KIM, a psychologist.
DR. GIDEON, an inventor.
HENRY SPRUCE, a judge.

GENEVIEVE BROUWER, REGINA REAGAN, CORALINE LEVINSON, } daughters to Levinson.

MARCO BROUWER, Governor of New York, and husband to Genevieve.
DOMINIC REAGAN, California State Senator, and husband to Regina.
SLADE, betrothed to Coraline.

DR. EDWARD GLOWER, a doctor.
ED, a nurse, and illegitimate son to Glower.
TED, a medical student, and son to Glower.

KEN WONG, a medical resident.

OZZIE, an assistant to Genevieve.

Ghost that says, "Poor Tom."
Ghost, of Ken.

ONE

SO HERE I'VE ARRIVED.

Borne by the tide.

Locked in a coma.

Without my own air to breathe.

Without an heir to inherit my fortune.

You'll remember what happened to young Tom Mariner, my hopeful protege, and me, that great wave that capsized our invincible vessel in the Queen Charlotte Islands, and deposits me here, now. Apparently to the intensive care unit at St. Mary's Hospital in San Francisco—or so I have gleaned, from my forced kibitzing, my wife having insisted it be a hospital closer to our home—where the nurses attend to my every need, asking me to do things I cannot, and alarms seem to sound at all hours of the night, disturbing my sleep. Never the more, I am still Steven Benjamin Levinson, son of Levi, possessing one-point-six billion dollars, however unleavened the bread of my current self-possession, to do anything about my means.

I'll tell you what I remember.

Tom and I were reeling in the largest king salmon ever recorded, a mammoth silver brick of flesh surely one hundred pounds or more, which would make it the largest by the history of such recordings, when I became overzealous in my estimation. Our engine took on more water than any could muster. And the same waves that wrecked and rusted the World War II transport vessel on shore wrecked our small fishing boat, sending me under wave upon wave. I struggled there, beneath the frigid ocean, to breathe, against those waves, then giving in, and have apparently partially suffocated—my heart preserved, my other vital organs supported by a ventilator.

Do you protest what I posit about my health? What you probably do not understand is that those who have partially suffocated are still there. Or "in there", rather, as I am. Or so I have learned. Though I cannot act, I can listen. Feel. Think. Remember. And am happy to recount what I have learned, to those who'll listen—to feel, think, at their own free will—as I await my fate. My assumption is that I shall emerge victorious, as I have at every stage of my life. In business. As a father. As a son of God.

But my fate is, alas, not mine to decide. Because of what they—my wife, my three daughters, and Danny—do not know. All that remains is my will, beholden to my final will and testament, which I only recently recalibrated, to exclude Danny. So that he might earn his own. Leaving my fortune attended only by the advisors and lawyers. To be divided between the rest. Until it is, I cannot rest, nor sleep. The hospital alarms will remind me.

Thankfully, I discussed my will with them before my accident. And had begun to discuss with Thomas my intentions for turning a few things over to him, that young man who reminds me of myself. The portion of my fortune I intended for him, that glimmer I believe he gathered, is why I imagine he visits me here at St. Mary's Hospital, in west San Francisco. The city's first. Started by the Sisters of Mercy by the 1850s.

There is a chance, too, I must force myself to remember, that I might awaken—fully awaken, from being locked in this somnolent awareness. A chance.

"What are the odds that he'll . . . ?" my wife asked Dr. Glower this morning, her voice urgent, the remainder of her thought, obvious. I can see her gray-streaked black hair, see the furrow on her always kind brow. A question she's been asking often.

"It's still too early to tell," he, the doctor I've never seen, responds. "Testing indicates a mild to moderate degree of anoxic injury. I recommend we remain patient."

What we seek within our first month of my ordeal is guidance, though the doctors, especially Glower, though leading the team, do not seem to provide much. They, too, are led by the same darkness I see. The same blind man's odds.

And what is ironic as I recount this to you is that I can see. And very vividly. While I know my eyes remain closed, and can feel the soft goop they place on them daily, I can see very vividly, beyond the constant red-dish black, the beautiful faces of my three daughters—Genevieve, Regina, and Coraline—the angle with which Danny always rested his shoulders, even donning his army uniform, so regrettably relaxed and cavalier; I can see my wife's breasts as she's changing clothes before our first gala, after I had made my first hit, speaking to me covered only by her slip, her body slim and elegant as when we were young, and my unquenchable desire for her, see the stages we visited with season tickets, that singular play of my obsession, see my life stark by pictures, however much these images are broken and torn and placed back together, overlapping, how they fold upon each other; I see the bright, vivid colors of San Francisco, its flowers blooming in botanical gardens, eucalyptus trees in Golden Gate Park, pink-cirrus-streaked skies, flocks of wild parrots, I see all things, the colors of the Sea Cliff neighborhood where our painted mansion rests, where we raised our children, I see the sunset over Ocean Beach and north to the Marin Headlands, so sprawling, containing so much space to my vision's darkness; when my sight has returned to its true, constant, reddish black, I then seem to always see myself in the mirror, scowling at myself, scowling at Danny and back in time, scowling at the future, which one has only time to see while trapped within the state I'm in. I ask myself what I'm scowling at.

But here I am, digressing. I need only someone to see what I see, and how the events of my life transpired. As all there's left for me is to make sense of them. So that the bow of my present might be wrapped before delivery into an eternal abyss, unwrapped and unwound. My trillion trillion pieces to be reconstituted, if so fortunate. Or if I am to come back to this Earth and breathe on my own, see again with sore eyes, recapture what I have spent my whole life capturing. These one point six billion pieces of silver. My soul. More than I ever needed.

And now all I need is an ear. So that someone might tell me whether I am ready to let them go. Like an apparition. Please come with me, just a little further—as my lungs inflate, without exhaling.

"I have decided to effectively eliminate Danny from my will," I said to my wife and daughters in the library of our home in Sea Cliff, that giant military orange art deco bridge observing by dusk-light, its sentinel lights twinkling like stars. I had gathered them—Genevieve from Albany, New York, Regina from Sacramento, and Coraline from Colorado—two weeks before Thomas and Danny joined us at Queen Charlotte. "He is capable of making his own money."

"Effectively eliminate?" my wife said, her tone urgent as in my hospital room, but more imploring. "What does that mean?"

"It means a small sum is set aside for emergencies. Only for the instance which he becomes homeless."

"Homeless?" Genevieve interjected. "You think Danny, our brother who just graduated from Yale Law School, might become homeless?"

"I haven't brought you all here to answer your questions," I said, standing firm and stern as I could.

“So what then, of us?” Regina asked. “Are we also ‘effectively eliminated’?”

“No,” I said with much compassion. “I have decided to divide the remainder between the three of you. And of course, your mother.”

“Steve, you’re acting erratic . . . You also just sold your share of the Fluor company and put all your money into an arms company we don’t even know is going to keep their contract—” my wife attempted, of my decision to support the long-standing invasion in the Middle East.

“Lia,” I stopped her, “I have, again, not come here to answer questions.”

The antique armoire opposite the oaken bookshelves, her favorite that she had collected, as so many other pieces, from colonial Massachusetts, seventeenth century France, seemed to glare at me, stern dark mahogany, for having cut her out of my decision-making. Its curvaceous front seemed to smile wryly at me. The rest of the room was darkly lit by low lights, the three of them sitting together on the couch where I had placed them. Lia stood.

“I beg your forgiveness, but I must ask each of you a simple question before I decide to whom goes what, and that is: how much do you love me?”

Before I share with you how they responded, I ought to prime the listeners regarding where each of their answers came from.

Genevieve, as I mentioned, I had gathered from Albany, New York, where she currently served as first lady of the state. Her husband, Marco Brouwer, was the first elected Hispanic man to serve this role, then at the beginning of his second term. He had come under some scrutiny for a transportation contract he’d negotiated with the federal government to build high-speed rail connecting New York to the rest of the eastern seaboard, whereby the bulk of the profits went to a company he had a history with.

Of course the gadflies said this giving constituted cronyism, and the papers were investigating. I knew he was innocent. Genevieve always blamed me for this misfortune, as Marc had come to me at the beginning of his political career for advice—not that I had anything earth-shattering to offer—and of course, for political contributions. This engendered in Genevieve both thanks and resentment.

Regina, who had driven down I-80 from Sacramento to be with us, had recently married Dominic Cornish Reagan, grandson of the former president, who currently served in the state senate and was rumored for a run, next election cycle, for the office his grandfather held before ascending to the highest office of the land. His middle name is actually the surname of his well-to-do family who arrived in California before the eighteen forty-nine gold rush, where they made a killing in mining.

Regina's winsome and warm smile masked an intense drive to prosper in life on her own terms, and I long felt her marriage was a springboard towards her own political career. For now she was biding her time, which as we all know can be dangerous. Believe it or not, Dom started out as an ophthalmologist, before entering the senate.

And finally, Coraline. My sweetest and most difficult daughter. While Genevieve and Regina had in their respective actions declared their love for me by marrying prominent men, Coraline had absconded to the small mountain town of Georgetown, outside Denver, where her fiancé, Slade, an automobile man, grew up before drifting to California. He has an uncle in the legislature, though is by my account a misfit, tattooed and pierced and the perpetrator of several unreported crimes. How they even met is a surprise, their shared fascination with Formula One racing the common factor, the track near Dixon the beginning destination of this fateful union.

I'll tell more about them as we go along. At this time I should say each by their own respects seemed to have already declared their level of affection for me. And yet I felt by bringing the issue into full focus that evening, I might understand whether I had made a mistake by my estimation. They spoke in the order in which I've described them.

"Father," Genevieve began, standing for her own emphasis, "I love you more than words can express, more than the values you know Marc and I hold so dear. More than your money, my health, beauty, or reputation, as much as a daughter ever could love—this is how much I love you."

This pleased me.

"Steve, this is . . . " my wife attempted to stop us, though her assent at my out-stretched hand said we would continue.

"Regina?" I turned towards her.

Regina then also stood. "I love you as much as Genevieve, only I feel her words are small. All the things she named—money, beauty, her husband—she definitely loves, as well, while I wouldn't even admit that I love them. Not even Dom. My love is only for you—pure and true."

The skin of my arms raised slightly at her last three words.

"And Coraline?" I raised my brow, certain that I would divide my fortune in thirds at my first two daughters' words. That is, until I heard my last, in a demure voice, remaining seated, say…

"Nothing."

I paused to listen to the stagnant air—and noted the acute smell of the book bindings.

"Nothing?" I said, incredulous.

"Nothing. I love you as much as a daughter loves her father and no fake amount more. You raised me and I love you as much as this requires. No more. These proclamations are ridiculous." She said, and then prepared to leave the room wearing her white, summer, floral dress, streaked pink, lemon, grass-green, and crimson.

"Nothing?!" I shouted, beginning to feel my blood boil.

But oh, as I recount these painful moments, I hear them at St. Mary's, in my intensive care room, as my blood pressure cuff inflates, compressing my arm, deliberate and slow. Bright reddish-black tells me the time of day is late morning, or afternoon.

"Pressures are elevated," I hear my nurse, Ed, say, unaware of what Cora had done to me then, what she was doing to me now.

Lia, Genevieve, Regina, the doctors, all spoke together . . . *wait, hold a moment*—yes, I do not hear Cora; and haven't, come to think of it, since I returned to this state.

"Give an IV push," I hear Dr. Glower say, the depth of his voice authoritative. He is surely gray at the temples. "Ken," he identifies a man I have yet to meet audibly. "Make a note."

"Will do," I hear Ken say, as my ventilator pumps. He sounds young and wholesome. I gather he is a resident, in training.

"Maintain positive pressure," I hear Dr. Glower say. "Saturations are good."

"Is he…" Lia says again, one of her lingering questions.

"Thank God Cora isn't here to see this," I hear Genevieve say to Regina.

"Right," Regina says.

"Let's see," Glower says. "Ken, go ahead and examine him."

"Okay," Ken sounds nervously assured.

I wait.

"Open your eyes, Mr. Levinson," I hear Ken say. "Open your eyes, Steve . . . Okay, I'm going to open your eyes …"

When he does, the slick goop slips, and he shines the light into my windows, and for a brief moment I make out vague shapes.

"Pupils reactive," Ken says. "Now, show us two fingers . . . Looks like he's missing two toes on his right foot. Show us two fingers, Steve!"

I try, though I believe the sedation has yet to wear off, and so my arm remains limp.

"I have to stimulate a little pain," Ken says, before my least favorite part of each day. "Open your eyes, Steve!" Ken shouts, before digging the pen light into my nail beds, the preserved nerves sending a shock-like pain up my arm, where my brain tells my arm to do what arms should do, raising as if to strike.

Get out, Ken! Leave me! My mind shouts as this pain peaks, feeling lightning striking an aged oak tree; then agony gradually subsides, an almost pleasing sensation giving way to the same aching that emerges in my branches when this ritual is complete.

"Withdrawal to pain is good," Ken says with the empathy of having caused pain.

This will be a routine to be repeated daily, my daily torture.

"He'd probably kill us if he were awake," Ken says.

"And maybe he should," Glower says. "There doesn't seem to be any progress today, which sometimes no news is good news," he says to all.

"Can I talk to you outside?" I hear Lia say, before their footsteps gradually wane from the room.

I hear a muffled whisper and Lia says something about Coraline. Perhaps she wants to save me the pain of hearing what Cora's doing with Slade, why she's not here.

"She has time—maybe she should go to France," Glower says.

Coraline is going to France? I suppose as good a place as any, as I rest here in this eternal disposition. If it were not for my active mind this hospital room would be a prison. Genevieve and Regina speak to each other.

"He shouldn't have blown his lid at Cora," Genevieve says, and the flood of what I said returns, my pressures surely rising again.

You ungrateful little brat! I had shouted at Cora, veins bulging from my brow, my vision of the dimly lit bridge like an ominous monster approaching. *You're getting nothing! I . . . disown you!*

My wife flew into tears to no avail—I was a dragon. And I hear her murmuring to Glower about my fire.

"That's just who he is," Regina says, hushed.

"And who's to say he won't do the same to us if he ever wakes up," Genevieve echoes her tone. "He always felt closer to Cora than us. And now she's fleeing the country. That pisses me off, that she can do that. This old man pisses me off, too."

"I want to believe it's just his old age," Regina continues. "But I'm with you. He never knew himself that well." And then, even more hushed than before, "I hate that doctor."

"Well, what are we going to do about it?" Genevieve says. "We don't have a choice."

"He's getting what he deserves, all these tubes and lines in this cubicle," I feel her touch my breathing tube, feel her gaze. "Maybe this is what he deserves. For us, let's think about it." Regina says, their footsteps then also leaving the room.

I am alone again, as the sick are always alone.

"For us, let's think about it."?

I made a mess. Though anyone would've acted the same, no? After all I gave Cora, for her to say those things, do those things? How could she humiliate me like that, in front of everyone I hold most dear?

Danny is eight-thousand miles away, in Kabul, and somehow he seems the closest of my children. Why have I pushed all love away? Why do I believe, did I believe, that my singular presence was enough? I want justice! I want them to abide the truth! I never cared if I was happy! And yet I have so much still to reveal about what I wanted. When I could still want.

As I lay here, naked, unable to move, unable to show anyone anything with my body, I have only my words. And thank God, a listener's ear. Eight-thousand miles! My thoughts have this far to travel. Those who have found themselves where I am are capable of much more. We'll see what lies upon the other side of the ocean.

I must travel the ocean, by a breathing tube and with my dry, lacerated mouth. As alarms disturb my sleep. And as my pure sight looks inward, into a heart that is torn and hopeful to heal. Without air, without an heir.

TWO

ONE OF THE MANY CURIOUS THINGS ABOUT RESIDING IN the intensive care unit, I've found in my experience, is the repetition. Everything seems regimented, routine. The chest X-ray every morning. The tech enters promptly at seven. The suctioning of the saliva that's collected from my throat, exactly on the hour. Blood pressures—oh, the constant compression of the blood pressure cuff—taken every fifteen minutes. My breath made for me at regular intervals, as no one really breathes, exactly every four seconds, fifteen times each minute. It seems as though the doctors believe that my humanness will be made better by their machines. As if predictability necessitates health.

Another part of this regimented routine stands that it remains run by the same people. Over and over. Ed, my nurse, Ken, the resident, Glower, my torturer, followed by Ed again to give me medicine—then Ed's brother, Ted, a medical student, fumbling around, then Ken again to correct Ted, Glower each morning correcting them all, Regina and Genevieve precisely at the beginning of visiting hours, eight a.m., Lia, my wife, for hours more than my daughters—then Ed again for more suctioning, Ted's tardy afternoon check-in, then Ken's, and Regina and Lia are back, usually with Glower and Gen, over and over and over and over, each day by the precise hours of the clock, ticking along without end.

However precise, and while I have learned what to expect, I can't keep what's next straight but for the shade of red-black in my eyes, indicating time of day. If they only knew.

And why is it that these hospital staff, and my family, speak to me as if I'm a plant or a pet, something they can just talk to? There seems to be something comforting to them, my lack of response, my lack of opposition. As if I'm their therapist. A respiratory technician told me about her divorce yesterday. A nurse's assistant about how her boyfriend never calls a week ago—she doesn't want him to call anyway, she just wants calls. While I don't mind their words, they are sometimes as alarming as the consistent chirp of machines, when they aren't humming.

For example, this morning Ed came and said something interesting.

"Steve?" Ed said first with force, as usual, seeing what I'll do. "Steve I'm going to turn your sedation off." For several moments he rinses me with a cloth. "Steve, give a thumbs up. Give a thumbs up, Steve!"

Of course, I cannot.

"Just wait until Ted gets here, Steve." I believe he means this benevolently at first, as Ted is the young medical student on the teaching team. Then under his breath Ed says, as if talking to both himself and me, and very slowly. "Ted will make everything better. He has to, because of our father. Don't mind me. I'm only a nurse, and his illegitimate child at that. He only knew my mother's body, a nurse before me, who's now dead. Don't worry. I'll eventually take what Ted has." I remain uncertain of the veracity of what he says. "I have a plan. Just wait . . . " he says matter-of-fact, drying my legs.

By the way he speaks I imagine Ed has slicked back hair, the coarsened countenance of middle age, perhaps a tattoo or two.

I hear Glower's voice in the hall, speaking with a man who sounds like another physician. His footsteps enter, the clopping telling me his soles aren't rubber.

"Hi there," Glower says in his care voice.

"Hi," Ed says.

"How are we doing?"

"Just fine."

"Any updates overnight? I had to come before rounds to talk with Dr. Eugene about his neurologic prognosis."

"No. Nothing to report. And, I haven't seen Ken yet either," Ed says, undermining the resident.

"You haven't?" Glower sounds instantly disappointed and angry. "I wasn't happy with his exam yesterday. It's time I report him to the program director, Dr. Cohen. I've been having problems with him for weeks. He documented that Steve has two toes on his right foot, when he doesn't." And then peremptorily, "He is no longer allowed in this ICU," as Glower's words build intensity from care voice to genuinely cantankerous, he ends Ken's time with me.

In all honesty I take credit. I believe my spirit banished him yesterday for the way he inflicted pain on me.

"What are you reading?" Glower then addresses Ed with the same aggression he's now borne for Ken.

"I got an e-mail from Ted this morning."

"As in . . . "

"Yes, your *real* son, whereas I'm only a…"

"I told you I'd only allow you to work here if you agreed never to bring that up."

"Well, I think you'd be interested in what Ted has to say about you. He clearly sent this to me on accident."

I can hear Glower's breath begin to build again.

"Here, let me see," his paranoia grows.

A pause allows me to imagine sweat dripping from Glower's brow, though I also imagine the coolness, the always coolness, of the intensive care unit, likely prevents these beads from forming. I feel an ache in my back before Glower explodes in whispers.

"*'I'll put him to sleep'?! 'Half my inheritance'?!*" Glower's voice is both intense and muted. "*So you resent me and he's a would-be murderous traitor!* You need to find Ted right now. Bring him to me!"

"I haven't seen him yet either. I will, though, by tonight. I think he's just trying to placate me. I brought it up with him a few weeks ago. This e-mail was intended for his girlfriend. See?" And shows Glower the salutation. I can tell Glower is rattled.

Suddenly, the entire room becomes alive to my blind eyes for the first time—I see the monitor hanging above me to the left, showing my heart's beating, the ventilator sitting like a robot to my right, the cabinets where they store the blankets to my left on the wall, the hanging hand sanitizer on the wall to my right, where they pump out alcohol that has become the most familiar smell, I see this as if I've left my body for the first time, but I am still in here; I see the windows of my second-story room, the sink where all who prepare to leave wash their hands to the front and left of me—with Glower standing there after examining me, silent urgency, standing there scrubbing as if the soap should wash away what he's now discovered. The emergency eye-wash station observing what I have gathered is Ted, his legitimate son's undermining of his will, to include Ed, his bastard child.

"They're going to do a continuous electroencephalogram today," Glower says to Ed, more calmly. "I want to speak with Ted before the day is over. This is his last day with us on the rotation. As for you and I, I don't want any of this to follow us to our graves."

Unsure of what he means, the clopping grows softer as he leaves the room—as he always does, abruptly.

"I wrote that e-mail to myself," Ed says, dispassionately, to me, proud of the shit-storm he's stirring. "I couldn't help it."

Moments later Ted, the object of his chicanery, clops into the room, late as usual.

"Well hello, Tom O'Bedlam," Ed says, like a snake.

Ted asks about any changes.

"Nothing dramatic," Ed says. "Other than how you've offended our father. Get out of here on your last day. You'll pass the rotation."

"I am afraid someone's undermining me," Ted says.

"Go to human resources to arm yourself—tell them. Go."

Ted says nothing but I can sense his fear. This seems to have been building for him, as well. While the blood pressure cuff compresses, his footsteps grow quieter until gone.

"Too easy," Ed says, before I am alone again with the chirping.

THREE

WHILE ALONE I CAN'T HELP BUT REVIEW MY LIFE. I suppose I should tell a little more about it, if what I have to say later will make any sense. And as we have no other place to go. I couldn't tell my listeners what I think about their reaction to my words anyway, though I am interested. Such is my plight.

My parents, Herman and Breina Levinson, chose the name Steven Benjamin, because they thought this moniker would fit better where they were emigrating to.

"If we'd had our choice, you would've been a Raphael or a Hans," my mother had told me when I asked why I didn't have any of the "old world" names.

They were from what used to be called Bohemia, but during the second War and what the continental shake-up meant for our people, my father heard about a job with the railroad business in Anchorage, when the industry was booming thanks to the military build-up. We'd have gone anywhere and might as well have, until a Russian friend of our family, Dmitri, familiar with the business, greased the wheels for our departure at the eleventh hour, what I understand was just before our "interrogation". And the rest is history.

That history is: Anchorage is where I was born and spent my first eleven years, and the love of the outdoors that led to my accident was bred into me. If you don't fish in Alaska, people look at you as if you're the strange one. Especially the bears.

We lived in a large house on a hillside facing Cook Inlet, with living room windows that faced what the natives call "Susitna", a small mountain that resembles what "Susitna" means: a sleeping lady. A beautiful sleeping lady.

The four seasons in Alaska—June, July, August, and winter—eventually got to my mother, however, and as my father had made enough, a killing really, by starting his own shipping company, to live comfortably, we became "hill people", relocating to Hillsborough, California. Where the weather is always sunny. And where the economy was booming, as well, by the mid-50s.

People thought I was strange there.

"Eskimo!" the kids in Mrs. Calkins's sixth grade class called me on the playground. And other nonsense, with their scrunched little faces.

"You have husky eyes," one girl, Maria, told me in front of a group of kids near the basketball court. She was my first crush. It was an innocent compliment.

That would have made more sense if mine weren't deep brown. Danny's are, somehow, deep blue. Real husky eyes. But I never let what they had to say about where I was born get to me.

We lived a wonderful, comfortable life in Hillsborough; we're talking people with basically gilded toilets and Rolls Royces that they only use to run around in, not even to impress people. I remember a kid from my high-school class drove a Porche. It made me feel poor for driving a Thunderbird. I knew we weren't poor. There are some people who are poor and don't know it; we were rich and didn't want to know it. Or there was always some unspoken guilt attached.

After Stanford and an MBA my father told me that I wasn't going to inherit his shipping business, which would have been the easy and cushy thing to do. Because of my expectations I had made no other plans and so was briefly without a job when I graduated from the year of business school.

"You're going to have to strike out on your own, as I did," he told me in our library one dimly lit night. Rather than do a family business. This news hit me hard.

At one point after graduation I had $25 constituting my bank account, and I wasn't sure where the next dollar was going to come from. My mother sent me money occasionally that year, when I was living in San Mateo in my hovel apartment, shuffling paper for a bank, welcome in my childhood home only on the weekends.

"As your father says, before Anchorage we didn't have a pot to piss in," she would say with those loving eyes. I wasn't sure how I was supposed to take that.

"You mean literally?" I would retort.

And so I did what most intrepid young men would do—I rebelled by returning to Anchorage, using a childhood friend, Ethan's, father's connections to get myself a job in the oil business, as my father had gotten a job in Alaska before me. But with a different industry that was about to explode. And without a war to spur me.

Somehow, over the years, however, and especially after Vietnam—which I'll get into later, where I was the captain of a swift boat at age twenty-five, and lucky to be alive at the end—yes, somehow as I watched my own fortunes grow within Alaska as a veteran, as my father's had, winning foreign contracts, hiring my managers, building a business over the next ten years, making my first millions—which have grown considerably as I told you—my resentment softened.

Somewhat naturally as a result, at age thirty-five I returned to California and married Carmelia, or Lia for short, my high-school sweetheart from the Beth Shalom house of worship, after we'd reunited in San Mateo, and with my newfound fortune we moved into a nice apartment atop Nob Hill, in San Francisco. Just down the street from the Delphi Theatre, where we always saw plays.

It was there, in San Francisco, that Danny and his sisters were born. It was his mother's decision to name our son Daniel, after her father. The truth is I didn't care what we called him, as long as it wasn't "Steven Benjamin".

"I want you to have your own identity," I even went so far as to tell him when he was eighteen and preparing to enter Stanford, as I had. The night before, actually, as I came in while he was playing video games. "You don't have to study economics and get an MBA. Do whatever it is that you feel you want to do."

Danny always wore a childish, innocent expression when he was either happy or didn't know what to do or say next. In fact, I don't think this tendency changed after he turned eleven on a family vacation to Montana. Anyway, he had that expression when I said this to him.

"I just want to make you proud, Dad," he had said, taking his eyes away from the television, where he was killing aliens or something. I believed him.

Making us proud was always going to be difficult for him to do, however, as long as he kept dating Elie Monroe. Not because I had such strong feelings on the matter, though Cammi felt he shouldn't be looking for a partner outside of the temple. Danny quit going there, however, also to his mother's dismay, the moment he turned eighteen, as well. She blamed me as I was always lackluster about it. Danny justified it by saying he was going to follow his "own personal faith," which to me sounded like one of those sentences.

In any case, Lia never liked Elie, and therefore I could never openly like Elie. I wondered if the situation had to do with Elie's natural beauty, which was undeniable and reason enough for me to understand why

Danny was fond of her, more than anything religious. But, of course, Lia would never admit to that.

When Danny decided to enter Yale for post-graduate school in the law, that's when talk of their getting married began to heat up. The question was always: how? How, with Lia standing in the way, and with me having to stand with Lia?

But anyway, as you know this went on for a number of years, and I'm not sure Elie ever knew that Carmelia and me were behind most of Danny's hesitation. Maybe Elie's optimistic, now that I'm here, listening to a machine breathe for me. Or who knows what she thinks? Danny's eight-thousand miles away, as I said, going door to door to try to root out the Taliban.

"Is this Steven Levinson?" I hear a voice from the hallway that sounds an awful lot like Elie's.

"Yes," Ed says. That scoundrel.

"Oh my gosh," I hear another distinct voice with Elie, that I recognize to be none other than Thomas Mariner's.

"Can we—?" Elie asks Ed, who doesn't reply. I imagine he ushered them in.

"He looks so—" Thomas says.

"—Peaceful," Elie completes his thought. "Did you lock our apartment door? The camera just said someone delivered a package," Elie says.

"Yes," Thomas says. "I locked it."

But hold your cocktail for a mere moment. I find myself asking—number one: *what is Thomas doing here with Elie, talking about 'our' apartment?*—and two: *what is Thomas doing here with Elie, talking about 'our' apartment?* It was my understanding that he had a fiancée named Anna or something that he couldn't finance.

"What are we going to tell Danny?" Elie lets out with emotion at the sight of me. "We can't do what we've been doing with his father in the state he's in? I feel so guilty…"

'Do what we've been doing?!' I think to myself. It is clear to me now: Thomas is making a *cuckold* of Danny! I hear the heart rate monitor increasing frequency as my adrenaline system still seems to work. The next blood pressure reading is, of course elevated, and Ed has to give me god-awful medication.

"Like you said, he'll figure things out. I mean, he *is* a soldier now," Thomas says, earnestly.

"I know. Losing me and his father, though, at the same time would be too much for anyone. Now that I'm here with you, I feel like such a terrible person."

As my blood cools, I also begin to think that somehow this makes sense. Elie had to look elsewhere. Thomas is a fine young man—anyone who meets him immediately senses this—even if my opinion of him is dredged through this, his behavior along the bottom of the ocean. Stealing my son's—I stop myself. 'Well, Steven,' as my mother would say—*well Steven, you had a hand in this, as well.*

"I moved here for you," Thomas says, as if defending himself.

"I know, I know," Elie says. "I know. My feelings haven't changed. But I told Danny I would come here to check on Steve, and after surviving the accident you deserve to be here, too."

They pause for what seems a long time. I hear one of them rubbing the others' back. It must be Thomas.

Sometimes life is a knot that needs to be untied, and retied. With what I've just discovered and my daughters in the state they're in, I feel my rope frayed. Overloaded.

This is also one of the benefits of being in the condition I'm in, however. You can always feel free to not react. Because you can't. And then your mind unties itself.

Which I must do, by returning to my regimented routine. These regular hours. Ed will come soon to clear my breathing tube. I am tired, and my thoughts drift. There is, I hope, time still for untying.

FOUR

"I THINK HE'D LOST IT BEFORE ANY OF THIS," GENEVIEVE says into her cellphone. There is no one else in the room I can detect. I hear his voice, probably from Albany, through the receiver. "Ozzie, my assistant, says he threatened to kill him. I'm not sure why."

I hear Marco's voice more clearly through the receiver. Can't make out what he's saying, though he sounds resolute, as always.

"Yes, and that's why I've decided to downsize the company," Genevieve says. "I'm firing half of management. I'd rather they take severance than equity when the time comes, which seems could be soon if what the doctors say is true."

Once again, the blood pressure cuff inflates as I feel the veins bulge from my forehead at what I've heard. I begin coughing and biting the breathing tube. The red-black is now speckled with white, moving spots.

"Hold on a second," she says. "He seems to be having some trouble. I need to get the nurse. See you when you get here. Drive safe. Bye."

Half of my managers!? So she can inherit more?! How could I have known the company I've spent forty years building would come under such attack?

My gagging allows me only to focus on itself, as I tell myself over and over again to remain calm, the only way this stops. Ed comes as I am successful, my throat's riot quelled—if only this choking could be a verbal riot against my duplicitous daughter…

I then feel the extent of my mistake more deeply in my gut, where they are pumping liquid food into me through my nose, to keep my poor, useless body alive. It gurgles up my esophagus. I feel as if I am dead already.

At times like these, when my mind has come at me faster than I can manage, and I know it is my doing, something strange has always happened. I am visited by a voice as if in an echo chamber. Similar to my mother's, but very different. This voice has always served as a means to speak elsewhere, sometimes to calm myself, sometimes to chide, but always to reveal the truth. It's how I talk to myself, I suppose. And I call that voice "the fool", because this is often what I am when I need counsel. As I am presently.

Here's a clown nose for you, the fool says, its voice androgynous, all other sounds, chirps, betrayals, drowned out.

"What for?" I answer.

For banishing the daughter who loves you, and the rest, the fool replies.

"The rest?" I say.

For never having more than you showed, speaking more than you knew, lending more than you owed, riding farther than you ought to go, learning more than you believe, leaving your wife and your brood, to chase fish when you have food; so here, take this clown nose, for it's what you've chose, the fool continues. With my eyes closed I see a face in a round hat, colors painted red, orange, and yellow, imparting this to me.

I want for a whip, as Ed wipes my face with a warm cloth.

I then hear another voice outside, which sounds like Ken. Ed rushes out.

"Nice jeans. Not working today?" Ed says with a hint of sarcasm, having been present when Glower said what he was going to do.

"I only wanted to make sure he was okay," the disgraced resident who tortured my fingernails and underwhelmed his boss says. "Sounds like nothing's happened."

The lawyers decide if nothing's happened, the fool interjects. *He's given us nothing for your clown nose.*

"Nothing can be made out of nothing," I reply. "And you are a bitter fool." I am caught between defending my torturer and my annoyance at the consciousness of my conscience. Surely Ken must have good qualities, as he wishes still to serve me, even dressed down, forced out of his hospital attire.

No, Steve. I am sweet. Or perhaps bitter. To not know the difference is bittersweet. You ought to know.

"Are you calling me a fool?" I say to myself.

When you gave away your fortune you gave away all other titles. President. CEO. Founder. Visionary.

"But I am still—"

Yes, you are still. Still as a rock. And you split a soft-boiled egg into two crowns, and in doing so made your daughters your mothers. Now your ass is dirt. I'll hold my tongue towards you and them lest I be whipped or banished. As Coraline was. For lying by telling the truth.

"What am I?" I suddenly feel powerless against the fool's reasoning.

A child. Your own shadow.

"But I have daughters . . . "

Which you will obey.

I hear two sets of footsteps enter the room, seeming to have fallen asleep—whatever sleep is to me. I wonder if Thomas and Elie have returned. It's the same silence as when they entered together.

"You made the right decision," the governor of New York says. "There's no way in hell he survives this. If he does, please tell him I'm not guilty and ignorant of the firings. What are those wires on his head?" And suddenly I am aware of what they did while I was napping.

"Oh dear," Genevieve says, her voice a lance piercing my auditory nerves. "He won't know a thing. And if he does, I plan to tell the courts how Dad treated Ozzie. We'll need him for the depositions. Those are the brainwave test wires. I forget what they called it."

"Genevieve!"—I want to shout through this tube which blocks and facilitates my breath, to which I've been condemned. My anger begins to return by pulses, so that I am thankful that I can't tell her what I really wish would happen to her. That she'd be sterile! That she'd know what a snake she's become! The ungrateful brat!

I have another daughter in San Francisco, though I fear Genevieve and her are in collusion, and that what I suspect only too late is that Coraline is my only true and loyal one. What an absolute mess I have made, and here remaining powerless by the state I'm in! As if an invisible wall separates me even from the opportunity to make amends for the crime I've done!

I suppose all I can do is answer their questions to myself, to think and feel on what the answers might be. To answer them so as to prepare for when I am ready to have all tubes and wires removed. Whatever they've placed on my scalp itches, and feels like some monstrous, insufferable plastic ooze.

"We're probing for signs that his brain is still functioning," Dr. Glower said before they connected them. "From its waves."

Functioning… I never understood waves in any form other than the ones that crash and carry people and animals to shore. Their relentless pounding. And if waves are what make us think and feel and reason and speak, then let them look at the waves in my head. They are as relentless as Genevieve's intentions to destroy my company, and I hope they look jagged and fearsome to anyone reading into their meaning.

More afraid I have become of my actions, of what I've done to Danny. In my heart I feel those decisions were right, encouraging him to go to Afghanistan, to wait and see with Elie. These were my intentions. And I believed they were good. My full support would cripple him. This is what I would tell Genevieve. What choice did this truth leave me?

Lia would unplug the ventilator if she knew the way I truly feel, as I have done everything to keep my true feelings from her. That I wouldn't mind having Elie as a daughter-in-law, even though she doesn't worship at the temple, that I feel I should have given Danny more for himself, and not taken by the form of trying to mold him in my image. And still, she must know, without my words. As she does.

This weighs so heavily on the remnants of my abilities that I am comforted only by the truth. I can do nothing. As the fool reminded me, nothing comes of nothing. And so what I've set in motion, by my choices, is all there is and all that will be. I am thankful only that my mind continues to process, that my senses continue to gather, and that my language remains intact. One has a chance at consciousness if these three elements remain intact.

FIVE

LET'S GET OUT OF THE HOSPITAL FOR A WHILE. IS THERE any place a human being would rather not be than an intensive care room? Any space? What confines us is only as limiting as we allow. For, as I am learning, we are always free to go.

Come with me, then, on my first saunter with Lia, after I'd returned. In Marin County. We've reached our early thirties and are growing fond of each other.

We had met, as I mentioned, at the Beth Shalom Temple of San Mateo, in high-school. I was an awkward kid, too bookish for my own good, but I was really hiding behind them, and she knew. She, too, was bookish, however much we did not identify ourselves as the "smart kids". Her father was a neuroscientist who had started some companies and played the third flute in the San Francisco Philharmonic. Was always returning home wearing a bow tie. While I tried to charm Carmelia with my knowledge of Joyce, James, and Jane Austen—though the latter was only to impress her. She knew.

"*Mansfield Park* is actually a metaphor for British colonialism," I would say, earnestly, quoting something I'd only read. While she demurred. We were supposed to be studying for a midterm exam on Realism, and she must have sensed I was speaking beyond my means. The fact that I asked her to study surreptitiously as a date also was probably not lost on her.

"It's actually a challenge to Victorian slavery," she said, authoritatively. The fact that she was allowing the pretense was enough to encourage me. Though she acted as if I was stupid and she hated me. In some strange way I liked it.

Fast forward merely a few years to my departure for Alaska, and you'll find further proof that she was resisting temptation.

"I just want to support you after what you've been through," she said with yearning eyes that said she wanted me to learn to take care of myself, again under the pretense that we were friends meeting for coffee before one of us moved away. I was still shuffling paper for the bank and a year away from being drafted to Vietnam from my oil gig.

"You don't know what I've been through," I told her. "How can you possibly want to take care of someone who's been where I've had to go, anyway?"

"Don't talk like that," she said, sweeping her beautiful and slightly curled black hair to the right. She is where Danny gets any of his looks. "It wasn't your fault."

"There isn't any fault to be distributed," I said.

"But you're better now. You don't have to go. Think of all the friends you have here. Like me."

Again, that word—"friend"—seemed fraught after all the years she'd spent keeping me at arm's length. There isn't anything worse for a young man than to be kept at arm's length by the woman he's in love with. There, I said it. I was in love with her. Somehow, I think she was waiting for me to prove myself. Which I was doing by going back to Alaska.

What she's referring to isn't something I want to keep a secret from you either. Let's just say that, when I was essentially kicked to the curb by my old man, and had nowhere to turn to, except for the five hundred dollars my mother was sending me every few months, which didn't even fund my apartment and food, I had a little nervous breakdown.

How disintegration all came about has been the subject of some controversy in the *kangaroo court of my mind, where I sit as the judge in clown shoes, with a gavel made of candy cane,* as the fool might say. All I know is that it happened gradually and then all at once, when I couldn't afford to buy dinner one night and hadn't slept for two days and on account of all the marijuana I'd smoked with this other guy from the bank named Evan, who always seemed to have some when I needed some, to unwind, how we'd stay up all night not really talking, more staring at things like that god awful Indian they'd put on the television just so there'd be something on the screen overnight, the time was when all of this was going on for consecutive nights and worrying about my finances and not really knowing where the next dollar would come from as I said, just worrying and more worrying without any chance of relief, and unable to ask for help, that I started to believe that there was someone who didn't have my best intentions at the bank, the words difficult for me to say who they really were, it was merely some figment of my imagination I suppose, the boogey man except every thought was confirming that everything was the boogeyman, but that's what happened.

That's what Lia was referring to. While my parents never knew, I spent a night or two as a resident of the local behavioral health center I guess they'd call it now, which is really a euphemism for what they'd call bedlam back in the fifteenth century. The mad house. The infirmary for lost souls. Lia was someone who I always trusted and so when I called her to tell her where I was and she came and got me, and would still talk to me afterwards, as she kind of knew what I was going through, though not entirely, that's when we really started to have something. I can't really tell you what happened. As I mentioned before, my senses were too high, my processing too low, and my language was a mess. As for the answer, all I can say is that everything kind of cooled down on its own.

In any case, that's what saved me in Vietnam. You see, when you've experienced some kind of internal chaos as I had, external chaos is almost comforting. And that's what being in Vietnam was. Nothing but external chaos.

Before I digress any further and on account of being reminded of how it felt when I drove that swift boat, and as I've told you a little about Carmelia and me, let's get out of here as far as we can, to that brisk morning in Marin County when the sun was warming our faces and the breeze cooling our bodies, and we forgot all of what I've just told you and walked into the tallest trees on Earth.

"They're so big," she said the typical way she'd say something underwhelming and because you had to take it seriously it made her point better than if she'd actually put the effort in.

"Yes, they are," I agreed.

We had agreed to meet to hike as a kind of official first date, after I'd returned from Alaska. I was flush with money. And still awash and a mess.

"You probably haven't been up here—"

"—Yes, I know, in years," I completed her thought. While there'd been plenty of hiking in and around Anchorage, somehow this felt more natural, even though we were closer to the seventeen million people living around the Bay Area than the three hundred million acres of untouched wilderness throughout Alaska. I supposed this meant I felt nearer to home, also.

"Well," she said, pausing, breathing more heavily as we started up a hill.

"Well," I echoed.

"I'm glad you're here," and like an assassin, she shot an arrow directly into my heart.

There was always this thing I enjoyed when I went hiking. And that was when you made it out far enough so that you only heard the sound of your own footsteps. I'd chosen this path north of Tomales Bay for that reason, too. I knew that if we went somewhere trite like Muir Woods we'd be hounded by people and kids yelling to their parents how big the trees were, and I preferred Lia's understatements just fine. That and the sound of my own feet. And hers.

"How long are we going," she asked, following my lead.

"If we make it up the next hill there's a spot we can sit for a while," I said.

She assented by not saying anything, though picking up the pace of her steps.

We wound our way up. Whenever I looked into the underbrush, I always expected to see a deer or an elk or people camping—I guess because I had so many times before. But that morning there were only the natural mulch and bushes with light fog wafting over from the water, with shadows cast westward from the rising sun over the tree trunks, making the forest look as if ghosts might live there, as well. It was the kind of atmosphere where you tried to avoid speaking, so that you didn't ruin it.

The next hill took about forty-five minutes to get up, steeper than I remembered, and the fog was starting to lift, as usual by mid-morning. I was starting to have a few memories from Vietnam, like the time we charged up a hill, thinking the enemy was there after we heard a shot coming from that direction. They weren't. I fell in the mud several times as we charged, like in a horror movie, where you don't think the person running from the monster should fall, except we were running towards the monster. When we got to the top and no one was there Ricky Blevins from Amarillo, Texas, began to celebrate the mistaken identity of the hill by singing our company's favorite Rolling Stones songs, the two that

I can remember being "Satisfaction" and "Gimme Shelter", the latter having just come out; eventually joining in a kind of chorus and laughing throughout. Because we were happy but also scared. In retrospect that was kind of stupid as we were sort of announcing ourselves to the enemy. But that's what we did. And we never figured out where the shot came from.

My heart rate would have been elevated anyway that morning in Marin County with Lia, both from walking and being with her, though there was the added lightning bolt of fear that I knew was unreasonable and could still control then.

"Are we almost there?" Lia asked.

"Yes," I said, trying to remember if this was, in fact, true. I didn't want her to think it was a long way.

The fog was completely gone by the time we came to the flat stretch of trail that led to the cliff where I wanted to stop and rest. She'd brought granola bars, and I had sandwiches in my backpack, as well as potato chips with a salt and vinegar flavor, my favorite, and a bottle of sparkling cider. She didn't know about it, just as how I'd read up on *Mansfield Park* before our 'study group'.

As we came through the clearing by the cliff-face I remembered it was almost exactly the same, with a small patch of brown, dry grass surrounded by sagebrush. Probably about the size of a living room. The breeze off the Pacific was cool and crisp and calmed the nerves that had been struck walking up the hill. The sun was patchy through the trees and only enough to warm us.

"This used to be my favorite spot," I told her, taking a deep breath.

She paused for a second. I'm not sure if she knew I was hitting on her, which I was. I mean, how could I not be?—though we were still at the stage of our relationship where a little guile and misdirection was necessary. Which she accomplished by not reacting to how beautiful a Marin ocean's view was. I knew she knew.

"I see why," she finally said, with a tone that acknowledged the atmosphere that most can't deny. If she could I wouldn't have cared for her. "Why did you bring me here?"

And like that we were back to square one. And fairly.

It was my turn to pause, both feeling the residual tightness from my back loosen and trying to open myself to the possibility of truly dating someone. At the age of thirty-five. I suddenly felt my stomach flutter, which took a second, and then announce hunger from the hour-and-a-half of uphill hiking.

"I brought some sandwiches," I said, sitting down on the brown, dry grass, hoping she'd forgive me for not answering her question. I was realizing that if I was honest, I would have to say that I was in love with her. It would be a stupid thing to say on a first *real* date.

Again I imagine she sensed all of this, and so only sat down next to me, cross-legged in her jeans and light yellow Gore-Tex jacket. "Good, I'm hungry," she encouraged me despite my awkwardness.

As I opened my pack, I began to wonder why God had allowed me time with such a beautiful woman as Lia—beautiful both inside and out—and what the meaning could be.

We each took bites of our curried-chicken sandwiches and returned to not wanting to say anything because of how much history we had together, and how calm and peaceful places like this were, with the waves lapping at the bottom of the cliffs. The reason I'd brought her here. And then I realized it was also the reason I'd brought myself.

Eventually I needed to say something.

"Lia," I began, "It's good to be back in California." I tried to stay general, knowing where I wanted to go.

"It's good to have you back," she ate a chip and took a drink of the sweet cider directly from the bottle. I could tell from her tone that I was definitely still in the "friend zone". She just seemed to be enjoying my company and I wondered if I should as well, or proceed where my heart and stomach were taking me.

"I think at this point you're my oldest friend," I said, suddenly realizing how stupid my use of the term 'oldest' was for a woman in her early thirties. "I mean, longest," I said, laughing softly and a little self-consciously to diffuse my mistake.

"That can't be true," she said, "What about Ethan?"—that's Ethan Helms, my childhood friend from Alaska who got my foot in the door with the oil business. He introduced me to his father's friend, someone I didn't know, who let me start on a survey committee for the pipeline after ARCO struck black gold on the Northern Slope at Prudhoe Bay in 1968. Perfect timing.

"I guess I mean oldest girl 'friend'," I said, immediately cringing at my second stupid usage in as many statements. In part I guess sharing where I wanted to go with all of this. A kind of accidental Freudian slip. "I mean, you know what I mean," I said, not knowing if she did.

"We never dated," she said, to my dismay taking the confusion the opposite direction from what I intended.

"No, that's not what I meant," I said, "I mean, friend who is a girl."

"I'm flattered you'd still call me a girl," she said, my needing presently to acknowledge her womanhood. I took a deep breath before responding, realizing I also needed to calm down first. Or my awkwardness was going to run this sneaky first real date off the rails. I stood up and took several steps towards the cliff face. Where it was safe not to say anything.

To my surprise she got up and joined me, standing there.

"You're my oldest woman friend," I said, gratifying her with another strange phrase.

This time she laughed.

"Thank you for clarifying. That I'd get that satisfaction," she said.

Suddenly, and uncontrollably, those feelings of fear from the top of the hill in Vietnam returned, at that word. That song. Not that it had always haunted me, though I guess my nerves knew what it felt like too well to climb as we had, the kind of breathing it requires, and my body somehow confused my mind into thinking I'd come up that hill with Lia to kill NVA soldiers when she'd said the word we'd sung, and there was little I could do to stop it after that.

As I didn't want Lia to know what was happening, that or it'd certainly be the end of any chance of us dating—I mean, with what had happened after I graduated—and so I simply closed my eyes and tried to focus on my breathing for a minute, remembering what someone had told me in the barracks when I was finally being evacuated in 1972 at Tan Son Nhat, and that was to relax and remember to breathe. I figured Lia would think I was either just as weird as she knew me to be, or that I was enraptured with what was turning into a gorgeous late morning that day in Marin County, in 1980.

I opened my eyes and looked over at her and she had hers closed, too, as if imitating what I was doing, and it was then in that quiet moment I knew I wanted to marry her. Again, that would have been ridiculous to tell her right then and there, and my nerves were still charged, another wave of paranoia sweeping over me, and I began to wonder if I could ever truly marry anyone. With her standing there as beautiful as I'd ever seen anything in my entire life, I closed my eyes again and tried to think of what I was going to do to come back to sanity.

I tried to sweep my hand through my hair and could feel my fingers unsteady and almost shaking from how strung out I was feeling, and so closed my eyes again and tried to breathe. Lia was seriously into the moment by this point and I only hoped her intuition wasn't keen enough to recognize that I was rioting inside, that my body thought I was in danger. Both for her and to fight what I needed to fight. Suddenly I became angry at myself with doubt, and thought I could just end the whole charade by throwing myself off this cliff, and she'd have always thought it was an accident.

I extended my right foot a little bit just to see if I was serious about it, and then suddenly felt a fear much greater than anything I'd felt in Vietnam, and that's how I knew I wanted to keep living. Right there with Lia. But I needed to play it safe, both with the cliff and with her, by taking it slow. And so I told myself to breathe even slower, and I took a few steps back. And by the grace of God or Shiva the feelings of fear began to dissipate. There was only one thing to do.

"Lia," I said, fully calm and opening my eyes, looking at her intensely.

"Yes," she said, looking at me with hers.

I took her hand in mine, and felt the pressure of her grasp as I leaned over to kiss her for the first time.

It was the most tender kiss I had ever felt until that point or will ever feel again. It seemed to unlock everything we had ever shared or wanted to share though were too afraid to feel or say, deep and abiding, with the promise of a building passion. Instead of those stilted or formal or sloppy kisses I'd experienced in college from girls—girls and not women—who were either too into feeling their class, entitled to my lips, or were so craven to "make out" with as many men as they could and that I was just part of the revolving door of sorts. Instead it felt as if Lia was sharing her lips with me, without urgency, without jealousy or envy or insecurity or superiority; that we were simply united for the first time. When it was over, I only wanted to do it again.

"I suppose you knew," I said, withdrawing. However coolly I could play back to what I thought obvious.

"I never thought you'd be ready," she replied, without judgment. With the same tone as at the coffee shop.

I took her hand again and this time pulled her closer to me as we kissed, this time more passionately than before. As a consequence I began the habit I'd develop of imagining large, distant, celestial objects when in such a state, so close with people I love. I closed my eyes and what I felt for her seemed to expand beyond the edge of the universe—into whatever the universe is expanding into. That there was something infinite and ineffable entailed within that moment, and I didn't care what the universe was expanding into, that I couldn't understand, but thought that that's where my feelings for her were going, and I would happily go there with her and that's where our feelings were taking us, into the infinite unknown.

Then as quickly as it had begun, it ended. We pulled apart and we withdrew into ourselves once more. I opened my eyes and looked at her again, sure now that we were headed towards a relationship. That somehow something inevitable was beginning. And I didn't care about anything except where it would take me. Take us.

While we're stuck in this room, talking, it's to places and times like this I wish I could go again. If only for that same, brief moment. I'd give anything.

SIX

DO YOU KNOW WHY YOUR NOSE IS BETWEEN YOUR EYES? the fool says, returning.

"Why?" I ask.

So that you can see what stench you can't smell—but as for you, the smell is all.

If only the fool weren't so perspicacious. In honesty, my condition is the smell of this room and the smell of my daughters' lack of filial devotion, I can't tell which is worse.

Yes, the smell of an intensive care room is often stale as I'm finding, and yet as Ed washes my face with a warm cloth several times a day, I am managing to keep the smell of my mustache at bay, as they can't really shave me like this. What a small pleasure this is. And the plastic smell of my own breath through the tube reminds me of my true aroma. Of all my heightened senses, this is my least favorite.

Lately I've been counting the things I used to do, of which I am now limited in action. Walking was so fluid. If I imagine hard enough, I can feel the pressure of my body gliding down from my heel to my toes and my knees bending, only enough; the joy of my opposite leg swinging from my hip, an endless pattern of forward transduction and my arms swinging carefree and carelessly. Sitting was an immeasurable joy, the base of my hind quarters planted on a cushion, my spine perfectly aligned to that "S" shape they say maintains good lymphatic flow, my shoulders back and down, my head tilted just slightly up, so that I could see through my glasses.

Your daughters use you so you don't recognize yourself, the fool continues as I reminisce.

"How?" I wonder.

In crab pots in the Bering Sea, crabs wanting to get in, to taste the food, claw each other, one over the other, to the top, like human beings escaping a burning building. They shall treat you as a crab.

I am too exhausted to argue with the fool. "I agree," is all I can muster.

You should've been wise before you were old, the fool makes yet another incision.

"Oh, why must I be mad! Why?! I hope that I am not crazy! Let me be sane like the rest of them! Let me be normal! Ride my horse towards sanity!"

I laugh at you now. Laugh at my departure, old man, the fool says, granting me a reprieve. *They won't be maids long.*

But I know the fool is never far. As far as I can be from my processing power, sensory data, and language. I hear footsteps, loud from my heightened hearing. It's Ed. Talking on one of those closed-circuit phones.

"Tonight? Visiting hours are only until eight. You're planning on coming soon . . . okay . . . then you should be okay. Yes, I'm involved in a situation with my brother, thank you for asking." He pauses while I recognize Regina's voice coming out of the receiver. "Dr. Glower can update you on the tests we've done. The brainwave test, the EEG, is still running."

He hangs up. Per the routine I've become accustomed to, he clears the saliva that's gathered in my throat around the breathing tube, and repositions me so that sores do not form where I've been laying for so long. Due to pressure.

"Your Reagan daughter is coming to visit you tonight, Steve," he talks to me. As they all do. "And Coraline called social work earlier this morning. From France. She's hired attorneys."

I've begun to hate the bastard. Even though I couldn't survive without him. It reminds me of how we can love people while not liking them. Or hate them at the same time. For Ed I feel mostly hate. With his scheming, as if no one knows. I know. And when I wake up…

Then I hear further footsteps, and the same high-pitched voice I recognized before. Ted has returned, as well.

"Well, aren't you bold," Ed says with insidious sarcasm. "If I were you I'd get out of here. You might survive this rotation, though he's after you now."

"I just had to check in," Ted again sounds out of breath. "I can't leave patients without—"

"—He'll be here any minute. I'll tell him your tardiness was my fault," Ed lies. "That I put you up to it. Let me at least tell him you showed up late for a week because I told you to. Let me do it in my effort save you."

"Okay," Ted pauses. I can hear the distress in his voice. "I'm out of here."

I could sense based on my acclimation to the ICU routine that Glower was near. And he was.

"What did Ted tell you? *Where is he?*" The angry boss announces his presence, about fifteen minutes later, here for his end-of-day, late-afternoon rounds.

"He tried to persuade me to . . . to . . . " Ed feigns his own distress.

"To what?"

"To get you fired." Glower's silence lets me know the extent of his anger, as he can say nothing. "He's already filed a complaint against me."

I hear Glower dialing urgently. "Martha, I want you to set up a meeting between my son, Ted, as well as Ed—the ICU nurse—and me. No questions. Just find him."

His voice sounds reasoned until Ed says, "When I told him he would lose this battle, he said he would sue until you're bankrupt."

"That—!!!" I can hear the anger return, hushed tones. "I've done nothing but support him!"

"I guess he feels the opposite," Ed says, matter-of-factly. His transition from feigned distress to coolness in the midst of such deception and what he intends to elicit from his father stirs my hatred of him again.

At that moment, however, and sooner than I expected—they must have been waiting in the parking garage when they called—Regina and her husband's voices emerge from the darkness, distantly and growing nearer. I am oddly at peace hearing her voice, and angered hearing his. This is probably because of how much time her husband, Dom, or "Dumb Dom" as I've ended up calling him, spent reminding me that he's related to the former president, as if this were compensation enough for his duplicitous nature.

Anyway, they're here now.

"Ed!" Dom says ignoring Glower and as if he and Ed are old friends, even though they just met last week.

"Senator," Ed returns, dutifully.

"We heard about the medical student," Regina says. "And he's your?"

"Yes, my . . . "

"They're both my sons," Glower says, sheepishly, concealing animus. "It wouldn't be professional of us to discuss . . . "

"No, absolutely," Regina inserts herself where she's not wanted. This is a consequence of having been around Dumb Dom too long. His intrusiveness rubs off on most people eventually including myself at times. "We heard and want to support you, Ed. Dr. Glower."

"We hear you're faithful to your father, Ed?" Dom continues. Again, they've just met.

"I am, as well as yours-in-law," Ed says as a true ignobleman.

Amidst this I hear the blood pressure cuff inflate again, and sure enough these people are pissing me off.

Yes, as a liar and a showman, Dumb Dom seems content eliciting positive emotions in anyone by finding what's important to them, then exploiting that with sensory data and language. Like I'm sure he just effusively smiled or gave a fake concerned look when he supported Ed. What Dumb Dom lacks is processing power.

"We're going to need to trust you if Steve here is going to survive," Dom continues.

"And we can relate to your situation," Regina says with equipoise to Ed and Glower. "My father rewrote his will and advanced directives before the accident, and my sister and I are—"

"I know. I'm sorry," Glower says, this time with genuine empathy. I can tell when he's doing his care voice. "I heard all about it from Carmelia and Genevieve. We have good social workers to walk you through what you might ought do regarding what his wishes might well have been."

"Thank you," Regina says. "I think we know."

They've hired lawyers, too, the fool fills me in.

SEVEN

I SUPPOSE IT'S ABOUT TIME I LET LISTENERS IN ON A secret. Well, actually, I can't right away, because if I simply said what happened—we're talking in Alaska—number one no-one would believe me, and number two I don't want the truth to change the way anyone thinks of me. I've already had enough of that, what with tubes coming out of my mouth and other parts and whatnot. Dehumanization happens fast.

To understand what I need to say, not about me, for starters, but about my father, I'll need to explain a few things about when I'd moved back to Alaska after I completed my Vietnam service commitment. The kinds of things I got into before I was Steven Benjamin Levinson, oil baron. Or whatever you want to call it.

While one might imagine times were always easy for me, because they've met me after I'd made enough money to essentially eliminate all discomfort in my life, there were actually more occasions in Alaska when the clocks were casting doubt. When the secret was the most uncomfortable thing I'd ever learned. Before I got my big break.

You see, most of the oil in Alaska is located in what's called the "Northern Slope", essentially a fancy name for wilderness that runs about one third of the way south from the Arctic Sea down into the mainland of Alaska. Until tundra and forest run into the Brooks Mountain Range that shoot up and divide the state. The railroad my father helped build and operate only runs as far north from Anchorage as Fairbanks, on the southern side of the Brooks Range, and so there needed to be a way around them for my business to take off. And that's where the pipeline I would profit from came into the picture.

Other than herds of caribou and wolves chasing them, and bears prowling the terrain in search of their next meal, "The Northern Slope" is essentially the place people are referring to when they call Alaska "The Last Frontier". And this is where I'd need to go if I was going to claim my spot on the opposite side of the oil spigot that became possible in 1968 when they discovered black gold at Prudhoe Bay.

The biggest town up there is called Barrow and has about four thousand people today, mostly natives living off the land and riding snow machines around town. But what I need to talk about happened on rails.

It was 1973 and I had spent the last year in Anchorage and after Vietnam essentially trying to calm myself down. I kept a roof over my head by giving guided tours of Anchorage on a trolley, as even though I was now a veteran, Ethan's dad's friend, named Stewart Bundy—Ferris's father, didn't want to pay me just to be on a survey committee for the pipeline that was only a glint in these businessmen's eyes. This meant a lot of traveling throughout the summer time as we needed to figure out the best way to pump oil from the Northern Slope south, so that black gold could be shipped out of Valdez and a few other ports on those massive tankers, destined to become plastics and petroleum products that would fuel the beautiful destructive things of the world.

For the time being let's stay focused—I feel the regularity of my breathing on the machine, fifteen times per minute exactly, is giving me some pacing here—on what I need to say about what I learned. About my father's time stalking bears in Alaska. Before I believed in chance encounters.

"Steven," the really truly massive Russian man's voice sounded deeply when I introduced myself in the passenger car, sitting down.

I was headed from the port of Seward, just south of Anchorage, to Fairbanks, where I was supposed to board a small plane and travel east to figure out a way for the pipeline. Basically from the Yukon River and south, through that area.

"I know that name," he said.

He extended his hand which could have easily broken mine if he squeezed as hard as he could. He was wearing a black overcoat and there was a woman sitting next to him with blonde hair, drawing in a sketchbook while a young girl, probably four or five years old, sat to her left, reading a picture book with Cyrillic characters.

We were sitting, facing each other within a six-seater, where our tickets had placed us. I was simply trying to make small talk. These are the kinds of people you make small talk with where I was born. Alaska is a place where they say the odds are good, but the goods are odd.

"What's yours?" I asked for his name.

"Vladimir Bugaev," he said, staunch, stolid, typical. The woman he was with was probably the most beautiful I'd ever seen. High cheek bones, thin slits with bright blue eyes, a waifish figure beneath a white turtleneck, outlining what was underneath, leaving little to the imagination. "This is my sister, Natalya. And daughter Kira." Natalya glanced up from her sketchpad and smiled, not saying anything. Kira didn't look up from her book. Natalya looked as though she was probably just a shade over thirty years old, and with his graying temples I guessed he was maybe a little older. I was twenty-eight.

"What are you going to Fairbanks for?" I asked.

"We live there half the year," he said. I noted their family resemblance by their aquiline noses. "We spend our summers in our cabin on the Kenai."

"What do you do?"

Vladimir grinned and Natalya smiled but they didn't say anything. In a moment I just kind of felt as if they were mean people, even that Kira was mean, and so recoiled into myself, hoping to not have to say much more. But then he spoke again.

"We run a guide service. Year round. Summers it's salmon," which sounded genuine.

"I paint away the winters, while he chases bears and sheep around Fairbanks," she said. It was late August and winter would start to arrive over the next few weeks. The weather was a fifty-five and overcast, normal Alaska summer day.

"Forgive her. She's an artist," he said, and somehow what was dark and mean a few minutes ago seemed to have lightened. I was having a hard time figuring these people out.

"Is that so?" I said, increasingly intrigued. "What have you painted? I mean, what are you drawing?" I was so flummoxed by her beauty, like I was towards Lia later in Marin County, that I didn't even really know what I wanted to ask. In fact, my communication could have been distilled into the sentiment *"I am interested in you."* Even though I didn't know if Kira's father still fit the picture.

And how could I not be? Twenty-eight and single. Alone and lonely, deliberately trying to make a fortune. And not doing a very good job at it. I could tell Vladimir was used to this kind of reaction to his sister when he looked away and grinned again.

"Something based on a novel by our great uncle," she said, without naming a title. I didn't know what she meant by "great uncle", like he was a great uncle or he was one of their parents' uncles.

"Oh, that's very nice," I said, asking myself if I should bring up *Mansfield Park*.

"Uncle Andre!" Kira almost shouted.

"Shh, Kira," Natalya said to her, extending her arm around Kira's shoulder briefly.

He asked if I was from Anchorage and I told him the whole spiel about California, yes and no. I asked him the same.

"Our father moved us here when we were very young," he said. Natalya continued sketching and Kira was turning pages, sort of reading with her hands and eyes.

"I'm guessing from—" and I wanted to say just 'Russia', as if that could encapsulate the largest country on Earth spanning two continents.

Vlad interrupted me and said, "Yes, we're Russian. Ethnically."

The seats were upholstered with a red felt material that suddenly was very soft on my hands, which were perched flat on the seat beside my legs. I looked out of the window at the passing small pine trees which can only grow so high because their root structure runs into ice that's not too deep beneath the soil. Billowing gray clouds were spread across the sky with patches of translucence peeking through. The dark green of the trees went all the way to the horizon, where the black-brown mountains shot up.

"Do you live near your father?" I said.

"No," Natalya all but interrupted me, a traffic cop as I was crossing the street into unsafe territory. So that I couldn't say anything further. "He's no longer with us."

"I'm sorry," I returned. "Mine's also getting a little older."

"What's your business in Fairbanks?" Vlad asked, defusing Natalya's recoiling.

"I'm on a survey committee for the pipeline," I assumed they'd know what that meant.

"Is that so?" Vlad's tone grew more interested, as he adjusted his posture. Clearly he had an interest for the enterprise.

I found myself wanting company that night, as I thought about my father a little more. The formerly healthy and robust man he'd been was slowly becoming a memory. I thought maybe I could commiserate with these people. Prepare myself somehow. And besides, I was intrigued enough by Natalya to forget the real reason I was going to Fairbanks, where thirty minutes would see us. Which was that I had no money.

"Why don't you join us at our cabin tonight? For dinner and drinks?" Vlad offered, sympathetic. I'd been afraid to ask.

I agreed, as I still would to things like this back then. While I'd been morose that morning, somehow there was a tinge of joy in me, even though the feeling ran only about as deep as the pine roots into the permafrost.

And my multiple intravenous lines.

EIGHT

"YOU SON OF A BITCH," KEN'S VOICE INTERRUPTS MY memory reverie. *Who the heck is he talking to?* I think to myself.

For the first time I'm thankful when I hear Ed's crocks rubber into the room, and can tell in advance he's going to be pissed that Ken is here. It's as though Ed has a whole tube of Pringles on his shoulder anyway. But then a few other sets enter the room and it seems like things are about to explode.

"What the hell are you doing here, Ken?" Ed says, condescendingly. "You're already suspended. And now you're about to be dismissed from the program."

"Try me," Ken says, defiant.

Glower's voice then emerges, charged, from the ether, "Coming here without authorization is assault, Ken."

"I just got off the phone with Genevieve's assistant, Ozzie," Ken defends himself to Glower. "He's fake. And a nitwit. A Trojan Horse. He says they're preparing a malpractice lawsuit against me. Against you."

"Whatever," the unevolved Reagan relative says. And suddenly I know Regina is here, too. "That's not true. Are you crazy?"

"Not true," Regina says. "Though I do know you're here without authorization from Dr. Glower. Which means you've committed a crime."

"Call the police. Call security," Dominic says with the authority of someone who's family has been associated with the law.

"You can't call the police on me!" Ken says, a cornered animal. "I'm here to do nothing but take care of Mr. Levinson!"

"From which you were relieved of your duty, correct?" Regina asks Glower.

He pauses, and it seems for the first time pity or mercy for his underlings have gotten the better of my doctor.

"That's correct."

"Which means you're trespassing in a hospital. Call the police," Dumb Dom says again, and Ed begins dialing dutifully. "You'll spend the day in jail."

"How about the night?" Regina corrects him, as even my own sense of justice is somewhat perturbed. As far as I can tell, Ken's big crime was caring too much about me. I begin to feel guilty myself.

"Can I speak with you outside?" Glower asks the former President's grandnephew.

"*This is bullshit,*" Ken says under his breath, clearly too deep into the situation to simply leave. "This will not stand."

In whispered tones, I hear Glower attempting to convince Dominic not to have Ken arrested. "*We shouldn't be sending a resident to jail simply for being on the ward. Maybe if he were a stranger who just wandered in, unauthorized. But I did this to Ken. He's otherwise been a good resident.*"

"It's already been decided," Dominic's voice is full and I can hear boots approaching.

Glower enters the room again. "I'm sorry, Ken," he says, as the boots are now outside the room.

"Where is he?" a brusque voice inquires.

"In there," Regina says.

And with a jangling of metal on metal the same brusque voice says, "Ken Wong, you're under arrest for trespassing," as the teeth of the cuffs click several times, and Ken is led out of the room, without saying a word.

"Coraline's coming!" Ken shouts before the ICU doors close behind them.

My heart rate monitor rings a sterile tone slowly. That I am cause for a resident to be sent to jail does not sit well. Or whatever I do now. Sit. Rest. Lie. All things I used to do differently, and yet now have no choice. At times like this I wonder if circumstances would be better if they just stop investigating what's wrong with me, pull the tubes, disconnect the wires, and see how I do. I'm ready to accept the results.

I'm too exhausted to care. What can I do to regain my strength, lying here for two weeks? It seems as though I'm sensing a jungle, the same feeling as I had when in the morass of my service.

She was so beautiful and so helpless. So ferocious. Her name was Camille Le.

We had parked our boat on the bank of the Mekong River, not long after the incident which led to us singing Rolling Stones songs like some mad choir. Our mission was to seize control of a surrounding village near Cao Lanh, South Vietnam, the previous territorial capital, with overall strategic importance for stopping what we imagined was coming over from Cambodia. Supplies. Weapons. Et cetera. It was a day so hot and humid you could both breathe and drink the air, and my twelve men, most not over the age of eighteen, were charged with charging this village near Cao Lanh. You could do that with twelve men. We were told the rush was possible, as the village had less than one hundred people, probably unarmed. On that sunny, humid late July day.

I'd discovered the Vietnamese people, the vast majority, weren't dangerous. In fact, most were shirt-off-their-back type of people. But we didn't know that with our machine guns and napalm and agent orange flyovers, the latter two which thankfully hadn't been deployed at that point near Cao Lanh. It was just us. I was twenty-three, the senior statesman. In my second tour in the marines. Captain of I-don't-know-what.

As we dug our way through the vines and thicket one of my men whispered, "You hear that?" The branches softly breaking as we slogged through still echo in my mind, my t-shirt soaked through long ago. "That's my future wife, taming tigers."

"We'll see how she does with you," I said, wanting to keep morale up. "Now shut up."

As we drew nearer we could see thatched roofs, a clearing, people whose ancestors had probably lived that way for hundreds of years and would've been content to keep living, regardless of our troops' invasion. We were freedom fighter invaders, really, and they were recently free. Living off the land and whatever small supplies they brought from Cao Lanh.

Which makes perfect sense as to why they greeted our aggressive bum-rushing the way they did, when we finally charged through the clearing, bearing our machine guns, kicking over carts, shooting goats and pigs, not the villagers, most of whom were simply shocked and cowered and retreated. They weren't armed, as we'd assumed. That's when Camille started attacking me with a bamboo cane.

She hit me first across the back so that it stunned and stung me. She threw the cane at my head, striking my helmet, and then began doing whatever she could to assault me with her fists, which I caught in my hands, subduing her.

"Don't shoot her!" I shouted as a boy called Red from Alabama fired a few rounds towards the sky to scare her away. The pandemonium of our entrance to the village had peaked and then simmered to the point that she felt comfortable attacking me this way. I knew she wasn't dangerous and couldn't kill me with the cane. "You're feisty, aren't you?" I looked down at her scowling face, both it and the gray long shirt she wore covered in mud.

"I'm Camille. I am going to kill you!" she shouted. I was surprised by her Vietnamese accent. She looked European.

"Calm down," I said, as she writhed against my arms. "We don't mean you any harm."

"I will kill you!" She kept shouting as I heard a few more shots fired across the village, which I hoped weren't making me a liar.

"Here," I said, and took a piece of rope, showing it to her. "If you don't stop, I'm tying your hands up."

She seemed satisfied and deterred, having made her point, and just started staring at me that way only Camille could. She couldn't be more than nineteen years old. "How . . . who are you?" I said in disbelief. "Where is your leader?"

As I was told later that day in Hao Le's hut, it turned out that Camille's parents had been French missionaries, until they were killed by a North Vietnamese hit that had come through when she was only a child. The town had raised her just the same. And I wondered if anyone in France even knew.

"They kill Camille mother and father. They come back two weeks ago and do thing to her. They will kill all us soon," he said, their leader, whose surname Camille had taken. An afternoon breeze broke the intense heat. His English was also good. Camille, traumatized losing her parents and by this, probably thought we'd come to do something similar. I assumed what he meant by "thing".

Somehow that seemed to validate our mission at the same time it made me go from being Camille's attacker to her potential savior in a matter of minutes. And while we were the ones with the guns, they were the ones with the food and the knowledge on living near Cao Lanh.

"All right," I told Hao, "We'll protect you from them if you'll provide us with food and shelter until we needed to move on. We have orders to protect you."

He motioned for Camille to come inside, as if he wanted someone's approval, like he'd adopted her. They talked it over in their language, which I understood not a word of, and then after a moment Camille paused, looked at me, and nodded. She was a beautiful apparition of this gorgeous, haunted place.

That night and for the next six nights we lived with the villagers, ate roasted pig most nights, some of the ones we'd shot when invading, which tasted sweet and salty, and drank both coagulated goat blood which was better than you might think, as well as a concoction given to us by a medicine man, made from the root of a tree, that gave us intense hallucinations. Strangely how I feel now, as if it primed my brain forever or something. During the day we mostly relaxed and smoked. Went on a few near patrols, finding nothing of importance.

On about the third night while sitting around the campfire I found myself becoming kind of maudlin, like I am now, recounting this story to you. With a machine breathing for me. I guess the reason I'm remembering all this is because I feel similarly trapped as I felt then, like what business did I have in this village with these people, half way around the world, defending ideas I wasn't all that sure about anymore? I felt as if I was just surviving, like I am now. And it was then, a moment of weakness, as I gazed deeply into those flames, that I started to have feelings for Camille.

"Come, sit by me," I motioned for her, curious. "Let me show you something." I wanted her to see a picture I'd brought of a grizzly bear I'd taken near Mount Denali, that I kept to remember where I wanted to return to. Maybe she'd think I was wild. I still did such things when I was twenty-three.

She sat down gingerly. "Oh, very nice," she said.

"Grizzly bear," I said, the firelight illuminating her soft, angelic face.

I guess I was looking for someone to absolve me of what I was doing. While I hadn't killed anyone to that point, a few of my men had along the river. The stupid killings you saw in a war, never any rules, fearful killings of the innocent, just a finger on a trigger for less than a second, no courts, no arbiter but God, who also doesn't always seem to care that you're there. You did it to yourself. And so if God wasn't going to absolve me, then maybe Camille could.

"You are from Alaska?" she asked.

"Yes," I said. "And California."

"Oh, Cal-ee-fornia," she said. Her eyes enthralled me.

"Have you ever been?" I asked, knowing she probably hadn't.

"No, but I want to," she said.

"What else do you want?" I returned, placing my hand in hers.

Things like this happened quickly when I was a soldier. There was no time for anything else. The cliche that there's no guarantee of tomorrow only rings true in a war, and so when I felt the pressure of her hand against mine, it's perfectly smooth and soft digits, standing up with her hand, taking her to be alone, there seemed an inevitability. To my sinful absolution. Though I didn't believe in sin. Not then.

Back in her hut she kissed me as no one ever had before, deeply, aggressively, with an almost animal-like quality. They were kisses that were begging me to take her, take her with me, just to take her, away from what she'd endured in the past weeks, maybe her whole life, and even at such an age. There was no reason in the chaos of Vietnam, only boredom and terror and fear and longing, and this was longing's purest form, without the prerequisites of time. *Take me*, her kisses said.

When our clothes had been dispensed of, she stopped my advance.

"It will . . . hurt," she said, remembering the word. "But I want to."

"Okay," I said, feeling her hands on my back, going slowly.

"I want to," she said.

"I want you," I said.

"I want you," she echoed, whispered.

What we did over those next three nights was the consequence of love, of circumstance, as I conjured deep and abiding reasons. I would take her back to Alaska. Marry her. Live a long and comfortable life with her. Care about nothing other than her. I had forgotten about Lia, forgotten about everyone and everything that had come before, that cavalcade of distant disappointment. I had lived an entire life in three days. I cared only about Camille. Camille Le. It was like I'd been drugged, my brain drenched by love and adrenaline.

"When we go, you come with us. Will you come with us?" I asked Camille, the week before it happened.

"To Alaska?" she said.

"To Alaska."

"To Cal-ee-fornia?"

"To California."

"You be my…"

"Your husband, yes," I said.

She paused, running her hand over my shoulder as we lay there together. Perfectly together. Feeling the sweat of our bodies cooled by a slight wind. Naked. Together.

"Okay," she said, and we kissed again that way for the last time.

The next week, we received a report that the North Vietnamese had launched an attack on Cao Lanh. They'd aggregated their supplies and skipped our village. Radio told us our orders were to return to the city to provide reinforcements for a convoy that needed passage out. A medical convoy transporting the wounded back to Ho Chi Minh City. I brought Camille with us, as I promised. Something that would surely end my career as a soldier. I didn't care.

As we crossed a field entering the city she tripped and fell. A sniper, aiming for me, grazed my neck and struck Camille through the chest, killing her instantly. It took three men, including Red, to get me off the ground and keep going. I was in shock and my legs were jelly, but I kept going. If we all didn't the snipers would've gotten us. One got Red in the arm. We ended up the last vehicle of the convoy, firing back at North Vietnamese as an improvised dynamite detonation destroyed the section of elevated highway we were leaving on. Fifteen seconds earlier and we all would've died. I was so overwrought about Camille I reached for a pistol to turn on myself. Red took it away from me before I could.

"Your girl got me shot!" Red shouted at me. "I should shoot you!" He cocked the pistol in the bed of the truck, aiming it at me, grimacing in pain—only to unload it before he could send me to join Camille. I'm glad he didn't. More so that he took the pistol from me.

This is where I've arrived in terms of this intensive care room at St. Mary's Hospital, west San Francisco. The callousness I feel all around me. I'll never forget Camille, as these people who have professed to care, my daughters, my doctors, have forgotten me. I might as well have been struck by a sniper, rather than capsized from a boat. Seems more merciful, if you ask me.

I am convinced now that I truly did love Camille. Maybe the first person I actually acted on it with. Maybe she was my first wife in a way, convinced me it was possible. That was ultimately to be another time, like the year before, after I left Stanford, as now, that I felt ready to pull the wires and tubes. See how I do.

NINE

OUR TRAIN PULLED INTO FAIRBANKS JUST AFTER FIVE p.m. The billowing clouds hadn't thinned much, and were no longer extending to the horizon, so that I could tell the sun would illuminate their underbellies when it descended low enough. This would also take a while that time of year, as at that latitude sunset extends well beyond dinner hours. Which is what we were headed to their place ostensibly to do. To dine.

"Do you eat reindeer?" Vlad asked as he entered the large, textured door made out of pine wood opening their cabin on the outskirts of Fairbanks, on the side of a mountain.

"Yes, it's one of my favorites."

"Good," he said. "We'll have reindeer sausage, potatoes, eggs, onions, all mixed together."

"Yeah!" Kira shouted again.

"Great," I said. And I meant it, as anything warm and free sounded good to me. Natalya excused herself to go upstairs, presumably to change. I couldn't help watching her walk up the stairs, hoping it wasn't too obvious.

The stairs were to the right as you entered the front door of the probably fifty-foot-wide living room, with a hallway that led down between the stairs and kitchen, which was to the left and open to the living room. I assumed there were bedrooms or bathrooms or something back there. It smelled like most cabins do, I think because of the wood. Kind of musty and rich.

"It's also what I offer my hunting clients," he said, motioning for me to sit down on a deep blue couch in the living room, which faced two recliners.

To make pleasantries, I asked how long he'd been guiding; to which he replied fifteen years, since he gave up on school. I asked how he got into the business, which he was vague about as he cut the potatoes. He asked how long I'd been in the oil business, to which I replied only about a year.

"It's been difficult to count, as I got interrupted to go fight," I said.

He said he'd burnt his draft card. Something about not having patriotism.

"Do you want a drink?" he asked. "We make our own potato vodka," which sounded cliched, but I was intrigued and didn't feel I could say no.

"Sure," I said, accepting a glass he'd poured. Apparently, they drank it on the rocks. When I went to take it from him his sheer size—he was easily six-foot, five inches tall, and two hundred sixty pounds—made me think he could probably drink the whole liter without getting a buzz. Probably had a liver the size of my leg.

"I want one, too," Natalya said, having come downstairs, wearing black tights and a light, purple hooded sweatshirt that again outlined her slender figure. It excited me again just seeing her.

Vlad let her pour her own as the pan sizzled, the smell of gamey meat wafting throughout the lower floor. When the food seemed stably crackling and Natalya had her drink, the same vodka she'd mixed with grapefruit juice, Vlad turned to us and raised his glass and said, "Za zdorovie—to the health."

"Za zdroviya," I butchered it, though seeming to ingratiate them both for trying.

"You should tell me more about the pipeline," Vlad said, highlighting the real reason he'd invited me, as he plated our dinner. There was a pinewood table across from the couch and recliners where he motioned for us to sit.

The truth was every Alaskan was skeptical-of-but-interested in the pipeline, and I could tell Vlad saw the same dollar signs I was seeing for it.

"Well, I'm working for a decent company," I said, taking a bite of the fresh reindeer sausage, salty and moist, still not trusting either of them enough to reveal the truth about my questionable-but-optimistic situation, with Ethan and I just having filed paperwork for our own company. "Who are mapping geography from the Yukon River essentially to, well, here. So we can build most effectively. Then we'll go farther south."

"That's so interesting," Vlad said in his basso, taking a bite of reindeer, followed by a healthy swill of vodka. "I know that terrain well."

"He does," Natalya concurred, eating more ravenously than either of us.

"I guide up that direction every fall and winter," he said.

"That's interesting," I replied, immediately realizing with this statement that I'd made a mistake of opening the door for him to help me.

"Do you need any help?" he said, as I put a big forkful in my mouth, hoping to think while I chewed. I too swilled some of the sweet, potato vodka, to loosen my mind.

I was going to need a good excuse to refuse after the hospitality they'd offered. These kinds of chance encounters with strangers happened all the time in Alaska, where people essentially relied on each other for survival. You made fast friends. I'm sure my brain was performing all kinds of random calculations based on my processing power, however, and sensory data—i.e. emotion—and I was telling myself over and over to calm down, with the help of spirits, which produced the following:

"Sure," I said, on account of Vlad's gentle nature, great size, seeming safety, and the general fact that I really didn't know what went north to the Yukon River from Fairbanks. "I'm relatively new to the area and I'm sure we could use your expertise."

He smiled wider than I think I've ever seen a man of his size: like a Cheshire cat with piano keys for teeth. It was as if I'd told him we were going to Disneyland in the morning.

"I like you more all the time, Steven," he concluded. "Natasha, what do you think?"

"I would better if he talked more," she said, as I felt the vodka begin to kick in.

"Oh, I can talk, too," I returned, grinning at her, loose enough to flirt a little. "What do you want to know?"

"I think I'll go to bed," Vlad said, sensing my flirting and visibly tired. If the vodka had any effect on him you couldn't tell.

I looked down at my wristwatch and saw that it was approaching nine o'clock. If I was going to make it to the hotel I'd have to go soon. I also didn't want to give up on my chances with Natalya. Though they were questionable at this point. Vlad stood up.

"Why don't you just sleep here?" he said, ringing music to my ears. "I'll fold out the couch. What time do we leave?"

"Six," I said. "I just need to call the survey committee tonight, to let them know I'm here."

"No problem. Just stay here. Use the phone. I'll wake you up at five. I'm used to getting up early to guide."

"Okay," I said.

But all I could think about was Natalya. It was the first time I'd felt alive since what happened with Camille. For the first time I was able to forget the feeling that it should've been me who died on that field. Maybe give whatever this could be a chance. "I've still got a little in the tank. I'll show myself to bed."

"Me, too," Natalya said. "I want to watch a little TV."

Vlad took our plates and placed them by the sink.

"Natasha," he said, looking straight at her over the kitchen island. "Don't hurt him."

"Do you watch *Gunsmoke*?" she asked, turning on the television, as I kicked back in one of the recliners.

"It's one of my favorites," I said, meaning it. "I watch the show with the same kind of curiosity I imagined the Greeks and Romans listened to stories like the *Iliad* and *Odyssey* when the traveling blind poet came through town."

"Is that so?" she said, turning it on, slightly taken aback at my answer. "Why is that?"

"Because it's the stuff of legend."

"Well, I like it because they're all immigrants. In Dodge City."

"I like it for that, too," I said.

She poured us another round of potato vodka. I sat on the couch and she sat sunk into one of the recliners.

The episode we watched involved a captured native who was clearly a white actor painted to look that way, kind of ridiculous if you ask me though that's what they did back in that time. He escaped their injustice by the end, as he hadn't really stolen the horse as they'd accused him.

"Well, I'm glad he escaped," I said, of the conclusion to the episode, where "the native" has to do some bad things to the white people, so you're supposed to not be happy for him earning his freedom.

"You have a kind soul," she said.

"How much of the series—"

"—I've been watching since I can remember," she overlapped my comment with her answer.

In those days you just watched one episode before something else came on. Natalya went to the restroom down the hall and I couldn't help but sneak over to the end table and see what she had been drawing in her sketchbook on the train. I was sort of mortified to see she had been sketching me without knowing it. The style was lifelike with embellished features, almost a caricature. My eyes were big and brown, my nose long and curved, my hair dark and curly.

When she returned over to the TV during the latter segment she turned it down. She was a little tipsy by this point and instead of returning to the recliner, sat next to me on the couch. I could hear its springs coiling as she sat down the awkward too-fast way tipsy people do.

"Tell me, Steven," she said. "Do I scare you?"

"No," I said, holding my ground, realizing it was better to put up a fight if I was going to get what I wanted. "Why do you ask?"

"Oh, nothing. It's just that Americans seem scared of us. Russians."

"There are plenty of Russians in Alaska, though. Hell, you used to own the state."

"I'm not Russian, though," she said. "I have dual citizenship. No Russian passport."

"So where's your other—"

She immediately grew closer to me, placing her hand on my knee. She did so as I imagined she had many times before and to men much more inhibited than I was in that moment. It was as if the vodka had smeared Vaseline over my eyesight, dulled my sense of restraint, so that my hand joined on top of hers automatically.

"What?" she said. "You like me?" It was then I could tell she'd done this before, but also that she seemed truly interested in me.

What I had thought would be incredibly difficult was now laid bare right in front of me, so much that I had a difficult time summoning the gumption to actually do it. *Kiss her*, the senses in my lips and my arms and legs were saying.

And so this inevitability, like a key finding its lock, gave way to my sudden leaning over, and feeling her lips on mine, the smooth and sweet roughness of her tongue, growing more intense with each pass, the leftover saltiness of the reindeer mixed with the saccharine vodka, our breathing only through our noses until the in-between breaths. And then she pulled away as suddenly as I'd initiated this sensual kiss, which seemed to last fifteen minutes, though I'm sure it was less than one.

"How much are you willing to pay?" She said, and again it felt like a police officer arresting me.

I thought quickly as I had when Vlad asked me about the pipeline, not wanting to offend her with whatever response I could summon to a question I truly didn't understand. "You mean—?" Was all I could say.

She paused, and then said, "Come on, you didn't think this was all about your stupid pipeline, did you?"

While I'd never hired or been with a prostitute, it occurred to me, looking back, how demur she'd been, how quickly Vlad had gone to bed, how what he'd said before doing so, that this could all have possibly added up to the situation I found myself in.

"Natalya," I said, trying to break through. "You're not a…"

"Only when I need to be," she said. "Now, how much are you willing—"

"—I'm not paying you for anything," I said. "You deserve much better than—"

"—Oh, you bastard," she said. "It's always the ones that tell you you're better than—"

"—Natalya," I said, "—you introduced yourself to me differently."

"I am everything I've shown you," she said. "But—"

"—But what?"

"But we barely survive on what Vladimir does up here," she moved a half foot away from me, and I placed a blanket laying over the couch on her, letting her know I wasn't interested. After what happened with Camille, I was too traumatized to open my heart so quickly ever again.

"Natalya, you don't need—"

"—Don't tell me what I need. I was brought here to your stupid country, my mother was left in Russia, and we never had a father. This is all I *could* do."

"Tell me more about that," I felt it coming in waves. Kind of repeating what a therapist had once said to me. Kind of dissociating.

"He died when I was five years old," she said, speaking soberly. "Volodya and I did whatever we could to survive child protective services. Fucking foster children."

"How did he die?" I asked, descending deeper and deeper into the waves of sympathy I was feeling for her.

"He was killed by a man in a hunting accident. His business partner took everything. The court gave us nothing."

"I'm so sorry," I said. "My father, his name is Herman—" I continued, adding the detail to show I was willing to get to know her better, "—was also involved in a hunting accident."

The story had always gone that my father's business partner had been mauled by a grizzly bear tragically during a hunt. When I was still very young. That my father had shot the bear that did it. That he'd acted heroically.

Natalya paused.

"Wait," she said, moving even farther away from me on the couch. "Wait," she said again, as if collecting herself, her thoughts, and her entire being, which I had somehow violated. Her eyes grew wider. "What's your last name?"

"Levinson," I said, still mildly intoxicated on ethanol and my growing, misguided sympathy. About to be believe in chance encounters.

"Your father is a murderer!" She shouted. "Herman Levinson is a murderer! He killed my—our—" and as she paused and moved towards the stairs, I stood up, as it seemed the only thing appropriate for how angry and emotional she was. "*Volodya*, come down here!" She shouted. "This, Steven Levinson, it's Steven Levinson, the spawn of Satan!" Her words curdled my thinned blood. "Get your gun!"

I'd left my bag near the kitchen and getting to it wasn't going to be a problem. Though, somehow my legs felt weak, as if she'd transmogrified into a grizzly bear herself, and was roaring me out of their cabin. She ran upstairs and shouted at Vlad again, and then came running down.

"No, no!" she said with maniacal eyes, "You're not getting out of here."

By this point I grabbed my bag and my fight or flight response was definitely dictating the latter. I heard Vlad rummaging around upstairs through the ceiling, and decided it best to simply begin running.

"I'm sorry, I'm sorry," was all I could muster approaching the door, not understanding so much what I was sorry for, only that I needed to be sorry simply in order to increase my chances at escaping unscathed.

Natalya rushed at the door and tried to stop me from leaving. "Steven Levinson, you're going to die!" She said, her voice as shrill as a trapped animal.

I couldn't really say anything, though, feeling the effects of the fear weaken my legs, the vodka now thickening my head, as I shoved her out of the way, hearing Vlad's footsteps coming down the stairs.

I bolted out of the door and down the steps in front of their cabin. And ran. I remembered the curvature of the road up which we'd driven, and reached the bushes as it began, as I heard the first shot ricochet off a branch above me. Vlad's steps on the gravel driveway assured me I was being pursued as I continued running, now faster than before, diving into the ditch to the side of the road when I heard Vlad's footsteps on the road. He'd killed many wild animals faster than me, so I knew I stood a better chance of survival by my wits. Brawn meant nothing to a man of his stature.

Luckily the brush next to the road was thick enough, and the sunlight beginning to wane considerably, that I thought I stood a good chance at surviving if I found the right structure to hide beneath. Another shot rang out and struck a tree about ten feet to my right as I jumped over several fallen trunks. At the third trunk I came down and felt what I had only felt once before in a high-school basketball game, and that was my right ankle twist without popping, so that a lightning bolt of pain shot up to my brain, the adrenaline the only thing that allowed me to continue after my heavy arms raised my frame up, the forty-pound pack feeling light as a feather.

After another fifty yards the adrenaline wore off and I needed to stop. The trunk of a fallen pine tree next to a grove of younger ones provided both a shield for something the size of my crouched body, and the small trees a kind of natural fence.

Vlad was pursuing me more deliberately, I could tell by the slow footsteps cracking smaller branches, and for a moment I thought he might have given up. But for the next fifteen minutes I essentially tried to hold my breath so that he could neither hear, nor more importantly, see my breathing, as I only exhaled into my sleeve, my lungs burning from the rapidly cooling air.

"Steven Levinson," Vlad said, drawing nearer, his deep basso sounding as sinister as my original sense of him and Natalya, "—we're going to kill you, the same way your father killed ours."

TEN

THE DAYS GO ON, ONE INTO THE NEXT, CEASELESSLY. I suppose the way I felt at that moment wasn't all that dissimilar to the way Ken and Ted, the legitimate son, feel right now. Hunted by Glower, or at least hunted by something that was supposed to be a benevolent force. Trying to disguise themselves with jungle muck. As the muck comes out of me, with only Ed to clean it up.

But as it turns out, even if it's our ancestors who are hunted, especially our most immediate ones—as Vlad was impressing upon me before I knew a damned thing about what they were so homicidal about—we have some kind of memory of that which forces us then to act.

You're wearing rags when you should have been bearing bags, the fool returns in earnest. Reminding me that I've born daughters who had a medical professional arrested while they circle me like vultures, lying here in a bed that has truly never provided me with enough lumbar support. There's no way of telling them, and it's as if I never made a dollar my whole life.

Fortune never turns its key for the poor, the fool mocks me. *And you're poor, having drawn Ken down the hill with you. He's packed in as it begins to rain, and as I stay, he's flown away, and the fool's no criminal, by God.*

"What on Earth are you blathering about?" I say. "I'll need a better answer."

You'll have your answers when you leave this Earth, soon, the fool says.

I hear clopping footsteps enter the room that I have come to recognize as Glower's perfectly shined hooves. And a few others.

"Show us," Regina says. And from this I realize Dumb Dom, the former President's degenerate, accounted for the remaining clopping.

"All right," Glower says. "But I don't want to set any unrealistic expectations."

"I'm ready to let him go," Regina says for the first time; and as she says this, I hear the sound of a cash register over her voice.

"That's a decision we normally want to make as a family," Glower says.

"Well, we're talking, and we'll likely pull the tube within the next few days. He's old enough. He'll never have the chance to apologize to Genevieve and me. And half the company has been . . . liquidated . . . anyway."

"Okay," I hear a deflated sound envelop Glower's voice.

"What do the brainwaves say?" Dom says, sounding intelligent for the first time his whole interaction in the hospital.

"They're *equivocal*," Glower says, I believe testing to see if Dom knows what that word means. "They don't say yes or no, but somewhere between. A few epileptiform discharges. Kind of low-grade seizures are brewing. Though better than they were initially."

"*Low grade seizures?*" Dom says, as if he can't comprehend such a term exists.

"Whatever," Regina sounds impatient, "—Just do what you need to do."

Glower pauses and I hear two steps approach me. He asks me to show two fingers with my right hand, and for the first time in I can't say how long I feel my hand move. Not voluntarily. Just a few digits kind of making meaningless motion.

"Good, good," Glower says. "Now give a thumbs up."

It occurs to me that he thinks whatever I did with my hand was purposeful, and so I probe the connectivity between my brain and my thumb, seeing if I can do what he's asking. "Give a thumbs up, Steve!" He says more forcefully, as if I might hear him better. He pauses for a moment as I again attempt to summon the connection to my thumb. Desperately, as if my life depends on it. Because it does now.

Alas, nothing. Not even the movement "I" was able to do before.

"I think we're getting somewhere," Glower says with his voice pointed away from me and towards Regina and Dom.

"Good," Regina says. "But that, what you saw, he still didn't do what you asked him."

"That's correct, but he did something he hasn't before."

"How much longer until we know?"

"Based on his injury, the amount of time he was without oxygen, which was estimated at approximately fifteen minutes, and based on the brainwave test, the kind of brewing storm, and based on what we're seeing, I'd say it's still too early."

"For Christ's sake!" Dom says, unironically.

"Genevieve will never be able to forgive him," Regina says, a serpent entering its fangs into my heart.

"Forgive me for what!?" I shout without words. And I again hear the monitors begin their electronic symphony. "You animals, you beasts!" I continue, feeling my forehead veins as I choke on my breathing tube, biting.

"See," Glower says. "More activity than before."

"He's in a rash mood," Regina says coolly. "And I still don't believe you that he can hear us."

I feel several lightning bolts in my brain amidst the thunder. That's the only way I can explain them, sharp pains up and down my scalp, and inside like an electric eel has entered seeking prey. They then subside.

"I'm glad we liquidated half the company," Genevieve says.

"I agree," Dom says.

What an absolute . . . *absurdity!* I think to myself. *I'll have you both imprisoned or worse when I wake up!* I attempt to transmit this message to Genevieve and Dom clairvoyantly—*do you hear me?!* I force myself to think, as if exuding the words transcranially, directly to the center of their dark hearts.

I can't think on them any longer as I feel several more bolts, what Glower was describing as "epileptiform discharges," I imagine. I feel helpless against them. A monitor on my brainwave test begins to chime. I hear his shoes clop out.

"Excuse me," Glower says.

"Let's get out of here," Dom replies, rhetorically. "Something is happening."

"He's doing it to himself," Genevieve says, without the least tinge of concern.

"I guess I could tolerate him if he gives up the company to us," Regina says with the same rhetorical tone as her husband.

Glower clops back in.

"I've asked Ed to give him more medication to cool his brain off a bit," Glower says. "Two milligrams of Ativan."

"Why is that?" Regina asks.

"His brain is getting pissed off," Glower says, his bluntness to calm what character, or lack thereof, he's seen in them. Another shock comes as I hear him curse.

"I agree with Genevieve. He's doing this to himself," Regina says. "What a desperate old man."

"Here," Dom says, opening the sliding door to my room, "Come on. Regina's right. Something's brewing. Let's get out of here. Close the door behind you."

ELEVEN

ZxZxZxZxZxZxZxZxZxZxZxZxZxzxxXzxxxzXzxzZXZXZXXzzzz RAGE! x RAGE! *X* RAGE *x RAGE!* SAGE! RAGE! x RAGE! *SAGE!* RAGE *x* RAGE! RAGE x *SAGE!* RAGE! *RAGE!!!*

mountain-black-brown-lemon-light-fade-bright-eye-sky-light-green-EYE-RED-phosphorescent-green-skyEYE
red—green sky x EYE! And blue black GREEN sky blue purple and green light green x phosphorescent green x green metallic sheen x pink cut pink then purple cut purple x hurdles hurdle the hurdle and My arm x arm my arm X disarm disarm disarm disarm

and legs x legs x legs x legs x pegs x pegs and pegs x legs are plegs plegs and plegs and plegs—plegs

x nickel plus nickel x plus nickel plus dime plus dollar the other divide bastard brothers
but dime plus dime plus dime dime x time dime time x dine x time time hour—time

x Danny is here x Danny is here Hi Danny do ante Danny do ante x quarter my arteries x far from me and bite tube bite tongue x blood and DANNY!

humble x bumble my money x honey my money x honey my money x my *head my head MY head—my head is dead x my dead head my head MY HEAD MY HEAD MY HEAD* x heavy x heavy x divvy divvy divvy divvy, my daughters live—divvy

"Push the Ativan."

Uncle you're sane, uncle you're sane, you've blamed and blamed and tamed and tamed the game the name of the game is YOU'RE to blame… Rhythm VIBRATION rhythm VIBRATION x station elation my station vacation, placation—x take me to a place where there's no trace of place x race me there where there is no place

Uncle, you're insane.

Lia Lia Camille Lia

catch me Lia Danny Hi Danny

Lia Danny Hi Danny

catch me oh OH Camille oh OH Camille

pink cut pink Lia Hi Danny Catch me!

x shots x shots x fire x shots x Vlad and shots x fire and Natalya and *my father shot their fathe*r x shot their father

x FIRE x FIRE x FIRE! FIRE SAY FIRE x FIRE x BURN and BURN and BURN

x OH Camille x Lia-Lia-Lia-Lia SAVE ME-SAVE ME-SAVE ME !!!!!!!!!!!! X should have

been me x see x see should have been me.

"Two more milligrams, Ed. It's what Ken would do."

".."

zzxzzzZzzzxzzx

"Load the levetiracetam."

ZZzxzxxZZxxxzzxxxxZZx

"........................" *XXXXZZZzzzX*

"..........." *ZzXx*

x the sea calm x bring me to hovel house x spouse x shovel this hovelhouse.

....

I the fool hear priests and feasts and brewers and tailors and suitors for your daughters and
right is might
X night night
my tongue x throngs

and fields, Albion
then time

time time
property of matter
time
property of matter
emergence
time property of matter
time, who lives before
Time
Cosmic fluctuation, uncle

Far edge

More sinned against. More sinned offense.
"Two more. Now the Depakote."
Hi Danny Shadow
Coraline x true Coraline x you
Shadowoman x France
Hi Danny Hi Tom man
Tommy Thomas take over my business Elie

Thomas Take over

……………..

Safe …………..
Calm
Now then

Life x beautiful

Vomit
Brokenclouds vibration
calm

And yes x say No oh will I say SO

Rhythm Vibration

Vibration
Harmony
X love pours through bright white light
Lia's voice
"Are you okay, Steven?"
Where is my arm?
"I believe we've broken it."

TWELVE

IS ANYONE THERE? DID ANYONE HEAR THAT? DID ANYone see that?

"Looks like we've broken the seizure," Glower's voice sounds muted, muddled, as though it's struggling through the air, coming from near the brainwave monitor. "Let's let him cool off."

To say that I feel tired would be like saying that the ocean is "big". An oceanic understatement. While I still have no voluntary control of my muscles, it seems that even if I had, it would be of no use. I need to sleep, and do so for ensuing hours, involuntarily.

When I awaken, the following day, and when I say this I mean 'day' as the next time I am aware of what's happening around me—it could have been a week or weeks for all I know—I am visited by the notion that my condition indeed could be worsening. Or could be improving. Isn't brainwave activity a sign that my brain is still alive?

Instead, my brain prefers memories of survival. They also quickly return to me.

After clawing my way back to town in pain, hitching a ride with another Alaskan stranger, I made my way to the only hotel I could afford—I was still buying my own rooms at this point, as we hadn't started collecting anything and the company was deeply indebted—and that was the local Super 8. My ankle had swollen to twice its size and already had dark blue azure discoloration that would transform to the purples and yellows and greens, over the next few days. I was glad to be safe. But have rarely felt more alone and confused.

What had my father done? I considered it now a necessity I really didn't want, either Vlad and Natalya were lying but what really were the chances that they'd make something of that magnitude that up? Strangers. A hunting accident. The truth was my father had told me a hundred times that his partner—who I presumed to have the last name Bugaev, I only knew him as "Dmitry" and he died when I was four or five years old—the one who'd brought us to Alaska from Bischofteinitz, had been mauled by a bear during a kill shot gone wrong. That he had acted heroically by shooting the bear although it was too late.

So I completed my survey with the other stooges from Fluor. If I hadn't clarified that's the name of the oil company with whom Ethan had gotten me the job. We actually found a decent route leading from the Yukon River all the way just east of Fairbanks, and it only took a few days and multiple acetaminophen—and a little whiskey—for me to be able to participate.

My ankle wasn't completely healed for a month afterwards, which I spent convalescing at the Captain Cook Hotel in Anchorage on the dime of Fluor's CEO who took pity on me when I'd gotten back to town. He knew a little of my backstory and knew that I'd be sleeping on the street if he didn't take me in. He'd seen enough homeless drunks of his day and either by pity or insight of whatever didn't want me to become one of them before my time.

For that month I had nothing else to do but hobble around the best I could—by then I'd ditched the crutches—wait for my next assignment, which was probably going to involve a trip up north again, *and* take on the part time job of sleuthing what my father had been responsible for. The thing that had most recently almost gotten me killed, too.

The problem was I didn't know where to start. There had literally been hundreds of thousands of guided hunting trips in the years between when this supposed accident occurred and then. As well as thousands and thousands of accidents. Alaska has about three-hundred-million acres of untamed wilderness and only about fifteen thousand miles of road. It wasn't like I was going to be able to quickly go where it happened either. My first thought was to visit the Territorial Fishery Service, like a Department of Fish and Game, where I might be able to get a lead on where accidents such as these were recorded. If they were at all.

THIRTEEN

DON'T TAKE THIS THE WRONG WAY, BUT AFTER MY seizure, I've begun seeing things again. Not the kinds of things I could and can always see, as when I first started talking—the flocks of wild parrots in Sea Cliff, Lia wearing her slip before the ballet or that play, et cetera. Also some things—maybe you can call them people—things I can really only describe as spirits. I wonder if it's an after effect of the seizure or if they're really here with me. Maybe it's just that the right parts of my brain got a jolt. Though I would swear to you on the Torah that they're here. With me. With us now. In this very room. Right now.

Ironically, the spirits are of familiar people who I know to still be alive. Not so much ghosts, as spirits of the living. Maybe I can feel them because they're all half-dead, like me. I see Ken Wong, the resident, now experiencing jail, his kind smile, perfectly combed black hair, above an immaculately pressed, long white coat, his stethoscope as it slopes to my heart day after day; and Ted Glower, the medical student who my doctor fathered and fired in a fit of anger—the one Ed Glower, his other son, my nurse, duped and denigrated. Who names both of their sons, by different mothers, after themself, by the way? Dr. Edward Glower, that's who.

I also faintly feel and see Thomas Mariner's, and his is getting stronger and stronger all the time, as though he's more resolved in real life. Very strange. And I can't tell you why as I'm not choosing to feel or see any of this. I see his pure face right now, so smooth and marbley-pure and blank and listening and absorbing, no trace of an agenda other than to relax and remain calm and sentient. Conscious. And then it's clear why I'm sensing him more strongly, his spirit by visions.

"Carmelia said we may be getting close to the end," Elie's voice appears. Smooth and clear-translucent as silk. Immediately I know who's with her. And he's more resolved. "Steve had a seizure two days ago."

"Have you talked to Danny about it?" Thomas asks.

"Not yet. He doesn't have access to the satellite phone until next Wednesday."

"You are going to tell him, right?"

"I don't know what to say. If I do and he's given leave to come here, then what are we going to do?"

"You need to tell him before he comes back. Give him some time to cool off. For it to sink in."

"For what to sink in?"

"That we're together now, and this is what he deserves for the whole time he strung you along."

"Thomas—" Elie says, and I hear her rummaging in her purse.

"Besides, what with your whole society and everything, there'll be plenty of people—"

"Thomas it's not that easy," Elie says. "A lot of people are going to talk and say a lot of pretty mean things when they finally find out. While we've been sneaking around it's been maybe more enjoyable for both of us. Though, give the hounds a chance and they'll sic themselves on anyone."

"We'll fight them off . . . together," Thomas says. "Like everything else. Nothing can stop us if we stick together."

"I suppose you're right," Elie says, I hear her assent as she's dialing. "You're always right."

I do not hear the same crystalline calm return to her voice. Several moments later, she begins speaking anxiously.

"Yes, we're with him now," she says. "Carmelia said we might want to see him before it's too late—No—No—she still doesn't know what she's going to do. Apparently the choice is either pull the tube when the time comes, or stick tubes in his stomach and a permanent breathing tube in his throat—No—Danny doesn't know yet—Have you spoken to him? Me neither. Okay, I've got to go," Elie says, hanging up.

"I can't believe you're even speaking to him," Thomas says.

"Well, we do go back a long way," Elie says of her relationship with Ferris Bundy.

"But you said he was basically a snake," Thomas digs deeper.

"He is," she said. "But even a snake deserves to know that their best friend's father almost died."

"They're best friends now?"

"Or whatever you want to call it."

"The whole thing makes me sick."

"Don't use language like that," Elie says with a tone that says she's thinking.

I don't know what's going to happen to or with these kids. I can't blame Elie. Danny did make her wait too long. And I can't blame Thomas. He just had his heart torn to shreds for everyone to see. And Elie has that allure that would make it difficult for anyone if she came on to you. And I can't blame Danny. Watching them, or listening or whatever I'm doing right now, is kind of an out-of-body experience as it is.

If I woke up, I would apologize to them all. Take responsibility. I clearly could've dissuaded Lia. Given Danny some more confidence. And then we wouldn't be where we are, with Ferris circling, a hyena with a hump for a neck, and Danny the lion out defending his pride while the attractive wayward wanderer, Thomas, has come into the pride. And even if Lia showed up tomorrow, she wouldn't know anything different.

She'd be listening to my daughters plan the destruction of the father they've come to resent while waiting on Danny.

FOURTEEN

AS I LEARNED MORE ABOUT THAT "SITUATION" WHILE IN Anchorage, it became clearer to me that I was going to need to do a little more personal archaeology, as well. Almost like I was told by Vlad and Natalya that there was a rift at the center of my father's heart. Like the San Andreas fault. Like a black hole. That I was then feeling in my own. I can't really describe what it is. Almost like an apparition or the same kinds of spirits I began sensing after my seizure. A kind of sadness there with me all the time. And I wanted to get closer to the center. To the black hole at the center of my Earthly soul. The fault that if I looked deep enough would show me the center. See if I could illuminate it.

I had a plan for how to accomplish this. First, I decided to follow the trail. A woman at the Fish and Game Department told me they only sold licenses, so to check the news archives. I figured there must be something there. If I couldn't go directly to my father and I couldn't go back to Vlad and Natalya for fear that I might end up with a bullet in me, then looking for the story as it was shared publicly would have to suffice. I believe subconsciously I was working up the confidence to go back and ask my father, though I knew he wouldn't respect me enough until I'd made my fortune, anyway.

The Anchorage Daily News building is right downtown, as well, not too far from the Fish and Game Department. Not too far from the Captain Cook Hotel either, where I was staying. It was a modern looking building even for the '70s with a second floor of complete glass. I guess symbolizing transparency. I approached a native woman working at a desk in front of metal detectors just after entering the revolving front doors.

"You'll need to leave your bag in a locker and show an ID if you're going to look at microfilms and request archives," she said with a flat voice.

In short time I was allowed through the metal detectors and into the archives, where a waifish woman, wearing a plain navy-blue suit, as well as a chubby man about my height with curly hair were working at a desk. I took them to be the archivists.

"Excuse me," I said. "But I'm looking for any articles you might have about a hunting accident."

"Okay," the woman said, as if for me to continue.

"It happened sometime in the 1950s, and involved shipping magnate, Herman Levinson," I said. "Of the Troy Company."

"What does the article say?" The woman led me forward in my bumbling.

"That's the thing. I don't even know if there's an article."

"That's a tall order," the man said through thick glasses.

And he wasn't wrong. It's not as it is today, in 2015, where you can search a good amount of newspapers on the internet. There was no internet when I was searching. We were going to have to physically comb a lot of material. I was willing to give it all the time it needed, though, if they could point me the right direction.

"Your best bet for today is to just look through the daily papers for the years you're interested on the microfilms. We can look for more for you. It may take a few days or weeks. The booths are in there," she pointed to a door to the right.

I entered a room with a lower ceiling than the entryway and was shown to a booth where I'd begin searching. Like I'd told them I figured the accident had occurred in the fifties, before I had solid memories, and so began poring over editions from around this time. There are a few bear seasons in Alaska but my memory is that the accident occurred sometime in May, during a hunt in the Denali National Preserve, which is an extension of the park north towards Fairbanks. That's all I had to go on.

The truth is I only had a hunch that it happened in May, and after combing through a few more editions realized the hunting seasons were both spring and fall, which would double my work. Instead of sixty papers to look through I had more like one-hundred-and-twenty, and felt the weight of this on my shoulders and through my back when it occurred to me. But I kept going.

I was lucky to have developed a tolerance for long periods of time spent sitting and focusing while at Stanford—not so much the MBA but as an undergraduate—and so a few hours went by and I was all the way through the one-hundred and twenty papers from 1950 when I was only five years old. It wasn't until the late October edition of that year that I found a trace of anything interesting. Though I did find something.

On October 27th in the Wildlife section of the paper there read a headline "LEVINSON TAKES AIM AT NATIONAL SHARP SHOOTING TITLE". And sure enough, the article was about a man named Herman. The text of the article read as follows:

> *Herman Levinson isn't an imposing figure. Give him a 25 .6 rifle and a target—some up to one-hundred yards away—and he becomes a man to be reckoned with. Standing just five foot five inches tall and of stocky build, Levinson credits his early life in the distant township of Bischofteinitz, Bohemia, for his tremendous accuracy with a rifle, which this past weekend has earned him the Alaska Territorial Championship for the sport of shooting. He claims he was preparing to battle Nazi Germany as a sniper while still a teenager*

and would spend hours upon hours practicing his accuracy at a range near his hometown.

This skill, however, was rendered unnecessary when an emigre friend to his township offered him a position with the Troy Shipping Company operating between Seward and Anchorage. Levinson now shoots primarily for sport, both hunting and competition. His victory over stiff competition has earned him the opportunity to compete at the National Riflery Championships in Montana in the spring of next year.

Grinning as he looks over his winning target, which he shot both in the bulls-eye twice and once through the same hole, Levinson says he is only sorry that there aren't any Nazis left upon which to exact his prowess. He'll take a dall sheep, moose, or grizzly bear as a consolation prize.

It goes to show that great things do come in small packages. Especially when the small package knows his way with firearms.

While I'd known my father "knew his way with firearms", I had no idea number one that he trained to be a sniper in Bischofteinitz, and number two that he had won the Alaska Territorial Championship for target shooting. It was interesting but still didn't answer any of my questions. Only raising more.

As it was the weight of the task in front of me was becoming more apparent, the six-hundred or so papers I was going to need to look through. And so, satisfied with my discovery, I returned to the waiting area, as I'd spent the majority of the day there and they'd be closing soon, anyway.

"I'm going back up north near Fairbanks again in about two weeks. Do you think you could have anything more by then?"

"Possible," the woman said. "No guarantees."

"Well," I said, "I'll check back with you before I go. And I'll probably be back some days until then, anyway, looking on my own. Do you have any other recommendations?"

"You might try the police," the woman actually echoed something else the woman at Fish and Game had said. From this I knew where my next stop would be.

FIFTEEN

MORNING FOR ME IS WHENEVER I HEAR THEM FIRST. I can tell from the particular shade of red-black that it must still be early, before any family have arrived. My head feels heavy, as though my seizure has rattled a jar full of water and sand, and the sand is still suspended, settling. There must be gold flakes found amidst the sediment.

"The whole things stinks to high heaven," Glower says to Ed. "When I tried to stop them from arresting Ken, it's like I became an obstacle. They wouldn't listen to me. Ken shouldn't have been taken away. Maybe sent away. But not taken away."

"They're savage," Ed says. "Or Dom is, anyway."

"Don't say anything about it to them," Glower seems to be formulating a large thought. "What I'm thinking. It seems like there's a good amount of fighting between the husbands, Marco Brouwer and Dominic Reagan. And what I really don't want them to know, as I spoke with Coraline on the phone a few days ago and have received e-mail correspondence, is that she's planning a legal assault on her sisters." His voice takes on an insinuating, sensational tone. "Whatever you do, do not speak with Marco Brouwer or Dominic Reagan."

I hear Glower's shoes go out. Ed approaches me, to place the antibiotic goop on my eyes.

"I'm going to tell them everything," his voice serpentine. "A wrongful death will get rid of my father. Then I'll rise."

Ken's spirit is with me. I see him for the first time. White and diaphanous, behind bars, an apparition of sorrow. He went into the profession of medicine to heal wounds, and has emerged wounded. But still a healer.

"Here, enter this place." He offers me shelter in a jail cell.

"My heart is already broken," I retort. "My mind is free; my body is delicate. A storm has visited my mind, on account of their ingratitude. Genevieve and Reagan have driven me mad in addition to my sad condition, an unconscious invalid."

"Fathom half!" A spirit resembling Ted, Glower's legitimate son, covered with mud and tattered clothing, enters from the right in my mind's eye, startling me. "Poor Tom!" He shouts having apparent knowledge of Thomas Mariner's plight from his time taking care of me.

Here's a spirit, here's a spirit! The fool, familiar with apparitions, as he might as well be one himself, goads my brain.

I feel boundaries have loosened after my seizure. As if it and the conditions of my daughters have made me perpetually drunk. I feel as if Poor Tom has daughters who've done this to him. The only thing that could.

"I'm going to open your eyes, Steve," Glower's voice enters from darkness. "I'm going to shine a light. It's going to be bright."

For a moment the spirits leave me, and the red-black becomes a deep maroon.

"Open your eyes, Steve!" Glower shouts at me, as if believing I will. "Say your name!"

"I'm like Poor Tom," Ted's spirit answers as the red-black returns to darkness, "who eats Ramen noodles and peanut butter and jelly."

"I wish you had better company," Glower speaks directly to me, with sympathy.

"The prince of darkness is a gentleman," the spirit speaks directly to and about his father's heart, though he isn't aware.

“You need to join us, soon, Steve, or I’m afraid it will be too late,” Glower continues. I resolutely charge my flesh and whatever is left of what’s inside my skull, hoping the seizure has charged it sufficiently, and that I can do the rest before my daughters withdraw life support.

“He’s gone mad,” Ken says behind bars.

“I can’t blame you for wanting to let go,” Glower says, strangely as if he can hear my innermost thoughts, sense my inner being. Perhaps he can, if I can see Ken and Poor Tom’s sympathizer. “Your daughters want you dead for money. Ken said as much as they took him away. I have a son, Ted, who intended to have me killed, and so who I sent away. But—” his voice breaks, “—I do love him very much.”

SIXTEEN

THE ANCHORAGE POLICE STATION WAS LOCATED ON THE Northwest edge of downtown, near the courthouse. Which was a stone's throw from the statue of Captain Cook himself, observing what he'd "discovered". It was raining the day I went down there the way it always rains in Anchorage and San Francisco, so lightly as to necessitate a light water-resistant jacket. But that's all.

I entered revolving doors similar to those at the Anchorage Daily News, and for some reason decided to go around in a circle in them before entering. Probably making the officer at the front desk think I was off my rocker a little bit. Maybe because of what I was afraid I was going to find.

"I'm looking for information on a possible murder," I said bluntly to the officer, bluntly as if to the very situation I'd found myself in.

"And what's your interest?"

"It concerns my father," I said, stoic, stating his name.

"Was he the victim, or—"

"—I don't know. His name is Herman Levinson. I don't even know if charges were filed."

"I should at least be able to help you with that," he said. "Shouldn't take long either. Do you have time? Sit over there." He pointed to a leather chair by the hallway.

When I sat down and sank into the chair which was as comfortable as it appeared, my nerves began to rise. My chest felt tight. Tighter than it does now, even despite the breathing tube. And my hands became clammy. My breathing was short and shallow and I felt a mist of sweat form on my brow. I tried to tell myself to breathe. I closed my eyes and was comforted by the red-black I would give anything to transcend.

Approximately a half hour later the officer emerged, carrying a cardboard box. His search appeared fruitful.

"Here's what I've got for you," he said. "Files from the Levinson-Bugaev incident."

"What do you mean 'incident'," I asked.

"Take a look for yourself," he said. "It's not my job to explain things. Though I do have to have you sign these papers," he produced clipboard, "that states I let you look through them. It's a closed case, so there's no restrictions."

"Okay," I said, struggling to swallow the lump occluding my throat.

I took the box over to a table near the entryway, and began opening files which contained multiple envelopes. I first found what appeared to be a police report. In the boxes of the police report read the following:

> MR. LEVINSON DISCHARGED HIS WEAPON AT A DISTANCE OF APPROXIMATELY 25 FEET, AT THE ATTACKING BROWN BEAR, KILLING BOTH IT AND MR. BUGAEV.
>
> THE BROWN BEAR MEASURED APPROXIMATELY TEN FEET FROM HEAD TO FOOT AND HAD BEEN PROVOKED BY MR. BUGAEV'S ARROW.
>
> STATE PROSECUTORS FILE CHARGES AGAINST MR. LEVINSON FOR MANSLAUGHTER. MR. LEVINSON STATES HE DISCHARGED HIS WEAPON IN SELF-DEFENSE.
>
> HARRY FRANK, HUNTING GUIDE, STATES THE SHOTS WERE FIRED IN RAPID SUCCESSION.

AS MR. BUGAEV'S CHILDREN, VLADIMIR AND NATALYA, ARE MINORS, AND THEIR MOTHER IS DECEASED, THEY WILL BE ENTERED INTO THE JESSE LEE HOME FOR CHILDREN IN SEWARD.

MR. LEVINSON WILL BE BOOKED INTO THE ANCHORAGE CITY JAIL.

My stomach sank as I read the details of an incident which had set the course of so many lives and ended one. Ended that of Dmitri Bugaev.

Doubts began to surface. Perhaps his death is what *allowed* for our obscene wealth in California, as my father then became sole proprietor of the Troy Shipping Company. Why hadn't a trust been created for Vlad and Natalya? And how could my father, a state sharp-shooting champion, a former sniper-in-training, have missed his target? Something as large as an attacking, ten-foot brown bear, when he could hit a six inch target from one-hundred yards? And instead, fatally hit Dmitri? Or somehow have shot both at the same time?

I asked for copies and the officer made them. What I had discovered had also convinced me that a phone call to my father would be necessary to prevent my consciousness from collapsing on itself.

SEVENTEEN

"THOMAS, YOU'RE BEING RIDICULOUS," I HEAR ELIE'S voice. They seem to be visiting me with more frequency.

"What, that I don't want Ferris involved in decisions about Steve's care?" he says.

"He has a good idea," Elie defends her ridicule.

"To what?"

"He's pretty good friends with a doctor in D.C. who says Steve can be woken up."

"You're being ridiculous," Thomas says. "Gideon is in hot water. And besides, the Congressional Committee knows about Ferris and think he's a fraud."

"It's new technology," Elie says, dismissing the true gravity of what Thomas knows.

"Lots of technology is all hype and—"

"—They've already done it in Los Angeles. Ferris says they're doing it over at UCSF."

"Glower is from UCSF, isn't he?" Thomas says.

"Yes, and he'll need transfer over to Parnassus. It's not far. You can see it from here."

In my mind I look out of my window, grimacing at where they're speaking of taking me. I know the Parnassus campus well, presiding over The Sunset neighborhood of the city, on the other side of Haight-Ashbury, adjacent to Cole Valley.

"What exactly does this technology do?"

"I think they send sound waves into his brain and somehow that wakes him up."

"I think you're just second guessing," Thomas says. "What does Danny think about this?"

"I'm telling you," Elie pauses, "Whatever Ferris tells Danny he's going to be on board. I know them both very well."

Thomas is silent, though I can hear his breathing, deeply and with urgency. That he moved from Chicago to D.C. to San Francisco in such quick succession gives me the impression that he is something of an animal in shock. An animal for making the moves. An animal for being caught with untrustworthy people, allured by Elie's beauty, allured by San Francisco's beauty, that evil that beauty can be when nothing solid or warm or loving lies beneath the surface. Thomas has yet to find something warm and loving beneath the surface of Elie and of The City.

"You told me Ferris was a barracuda," Thomas says.

"He is. But even barracudas have good ideas sometimes. What if Steve wakes up and we can settle a few things?"

"What, like you replacing Danny with me, and Steve replacing Danny with me when it comes to—?"

"—You don't know if that's what he was going to do on the boat before this happened," Elie says.

"Well, if it was, then that's why I'm here, and why I'm as good as dead anyway. Danny's a soldier now and I know what soldiers do to their enemies. I feel so guilty," Thomas says.

It's the qualities that lie beneath the veneer that Danny lacks. That Thomas possesses. And so in a strong sense, I am pleased that Elie has jettisoned Danny for Thomas's favor. It both frees Danny and provides me the obligation to pass the very thing that will perpetuate his indecisiveness—my profitable businesses—along to Thomas. If

Danny had just had the courage to break from his mother and propose to Elie, none of this would've come to pass.

"We're all as good as dead eventually, anyway," Elie says, a rare show of the nihilism she's learned from the same veneer holding Danny back.

"But what happens before still means something," Thomas says.

Words after my heart.

EIGHTEEN

"YOU CAN STAY IN MY HOUSE IN MARIN, KEN," GLOWER'S voice awakens me.

The red-black says it's afternoon, and my eyes are burning. Now, while I can't prove it, before this moment and when half-asleep I believe I've also just heard Dominic and Ed colluding, developing closer allegiance, and Dumb Dom asking Ed to tell Regina about Coraline's plans.

"At least until this is sorted out. I'm sorry for what they did to you, Ken, arresting you. I feel responsible. Please, take me up on this. I know you lost your apartment. I want to make it up to you. Come to the hospital today if you want. You're being re-instated."

Ken seems appeased and after salutations they hang up. Glower appears to be offering Ken's freed ghost residence in his weekend home. Appeasement to avoid a lawsuit. Though the threat looms.

Is a madman a worker or a gentleman? The fool interrupts my peace.

"I am a king!" I retort, angry that my conscience has disturbed me. "I provided security to my minions. I sought territory through mergers and acquisitions. Others cleaned up my messes."

You are a mad worker to behold Danny a gentleman.

"I *don't* consider Danny a gentleman," I say. "I must now arraign my daughters for their crimes."

"The fiend is biting my ass," Ted's diaphanous ghost, who said 'Poor Tom!', appears haggard before me wearing tattered clothes. With phosphorescent blue eyes. What have his daughters done to him?

Don't trust the tameness of the wolf I am, or the boy in Afghanistan who loves you, uncle, nor the whore's promises, the fool says.

"Come, both of you," I say to my conscience and Ted's ghost. "Sit here while I place my daughters on trial. Wear a black robe, sir."

"Sit down," Ken's ghost appears, diaphanous and side by side Ted's, out of the cell, in a white coat with perfectly combed hair. "Just lay in bed."

"I am in bed! You fool! You rightful prisoner!" I shout, as the veins in my forehead bulge and the ventilator chirps. "I will try Genevieve for her lack of filial devotion," I say, exhaling involuntarily through the tube. "Is your name Genevieve?" I ask of the ventilator. "And there is Regina's anatomy! We'll find what's in her heart!" I say to the heart rate monitor.

"You've lost your mind," Ted's ghost says with laser eyes. "More than Poor Tom. Those are your room ornaments."

"My dogs! Troy, Blanco, Sweetheart!" I say, as I see my mastiff, greyhound, and husky occupy our backyard facing the Bridge in Sea Cliff, my monitors beginning a chorus.

"Go to sleep," Ted, dressed in tatters, says. "Ferris has plans for you. To wake you up. You'll need to sleep first."

"I'll wake now! Change your clothes!" I say. "We'll have dinner in the morning!" My delirium takes hold. "Or I'll sleep," losing consciousness for a moment, the monitors continue their concert.

"Rest," Ken says. "Glower's coming." And then his spirit vanishes.

And I'll go to bed at noon, the fool says.

I hear two sets of footsteps enter the room.

"He's pissed off right now," Glower says to whomever's with him, for the first time acknowledging my presence. "The last time I truly examined him he appeared to purposefully move his right arm."

"Sounds like progress," I hear Ken's mortal voice, no longer a spirit.

"But his family, since the seizure, are preparing to withdraw care, what I believe to be prematurely. Ed knows though I'm not sure who else. And yesterday I had a conversation with Steve's son's girlfriend, Elie, who told me that Danny wants him transferred to UCSF for ultrasonic thalamic stimulation. They want to do everything."

"I've heard of it," Ken says.

"It's a fairly new technique. As you know the thalamus is a center of consciousness, and this is one way of turning it back on. It's worked for several patients in Los Angeles. I feel if we proceed with Danny's wishes, there's no way Carmelia will withdraw."

"Is there an advanced directive?" Ken asks, a good resident.

"There is, and it says he wants 'all possible interventions until there is no hope of meaningful recovery.' And ultrasonic thalamic stimulation is a possible intervention."

"So we're going to UCSF?"

"We both have privileges over there. So yes."

"I'll arrange the transfer."

"Wait, look," Glower says as for the first time I can make out of the red-black three- dimensional shapes, living ghosts themselves, the shape of their shadows. I focus my eyes on them. "He's tracking!" Glower sounds like he's just won the lottery.

"Steve!" Ken says, and I can see the contours of his head, an oblong shape, his perfectly combed hair. "You're right!"

"Steve!" Glower shouts at me. "Give us a thumbs up with your right hand," as I anticipate that it will work this time. "Show us two fingers!" And with all the might of my brain I try to connect the circuit. To spontaneously move.

"Steve?" Ken says, as the shadows begins to fade again to blackness.

"Give us a thumbs up," Glower's voice has tempered, with my right hand held by his.

Alas, I remain unable. The monitors return to their normal, sterile states.

"He definitely tracked us for a moment," Glower says. "It's probably more urgent than ever that we get him over to Parnassus, to the eleventh floor."

"Let me make a few phone calls," Ken says.

NINETEEN

"DAD, I NEED TO TALK TO YOU," I REHEARSED TO MYSELF, pacing in the hotel room. The day had remained gray and rainy since leaving the police station. "Dad, I have some difficult questions to ask you," I repeated, holding the receiver and hearing the dial tone to build kinesthetic memory. To make sure what I have to say isn't foiled by any physical object.

When I came to Alaska, I hadn't expected to happen upon my father's history there. It was supposed to be my endeavor. And mine alone. My fortune made. In spite of his decisions. Which were less than kind. But here I was, feeling almost out-of-body. As though the truth was waiting somewhere over one of the mountains I saw below low-hanging clouds. Or on the other end of the receiver. There was nothing left except to dial.

"Hello," he said with a low voice. Still powerful despite his years. He'd just turned sixty.

"Dad," I said, before my voice caught in my throat.

"Hello?" He said again, as if he knew it was me but didn't know why I was calling.

"Dad, this is Steve," I said. "Dad, I need to talk to you."

"Where are you, Steven?" he said, his voice softening.

"In Anchorage."

"Oh, I thought you'd be in Fairbanks."

"I was. I mean, that's what I need—Dad, I have some questions for you."

"Okay," he said staunchly.

I took another shallow breath and then a deeper one, summoning what I needed to say.

"Dad," I continued, "were you a competitive sharp-shooter?"

"A sharp-shooter?"

"Like, didn't you, or anyway, I found some articles about your winning the Alaska championship for riflery. In the early 1950s."

Silence.

"And, I was just curious, did you compete for nationals? Were you training to be a sniper before you left the old country?"

Still, he said nothing, and I began to wonder if he'd hung up.

"Dad?"

"Steven, where are you getting this information?"

"I went to the Anchorage Daily News. They let me look at—"

"—Why did you go to the Anchorage Daily News?"

"To, well . . . " The image of Vlad's breath as he hunted me flashed in my mind. "I met the Bugaevs."

He immediately hung up. The moment he did was jarring. I called again twice before my mother picked up after five rings.

"Hello?"

"Mom," I said.

"Hello?"

"Mom, it's me, Steven, your son."

"Steven!" she said with the excitement of two months without speaking to me.

"Mom, I'm doing fine," I tried to take care of what I knew she'd ask about quickly. "I'm staying at the Captain Cook until the next survey, probably south of Fairbanks. In about two weeks. We already made it from the Yukon River just east of Fairbanks. I've got a loan promised for some rigs from Bank of the Northwest's investment division. I'm starting a company with Ethan, who's out surveying presently. We're going to do fine. But I called to ask Dad some questions."

"Well, I'm so happy, Steven," she said. "Are you wearing enough layers when you're out there?"

"Yes, mom, I'm dressing warm."

"And not smoking cigars?" She always asked since seeing me smoke one in California that I'd gotten for a poker tournament.

"No cigars. No alcohol really either. Mom, I called to ask Dad a few important questions."

The sound of her voice softened my anxiety, as always. Except I could feel the confusion and disconnect of my mind and body as my heart continued to race and my palms again clammed up, at what I knew I needed to pry out of my father.

"Okay, I'll get him," she said, leaving the receiver so that I could hear a few barks from their mutt, Toby. After several minutes I heard the receiver leave whatever it was resting on.

"Steven," my father said with a controlling tone as if to steamroll me. "You're not to speak of the Bugaevs ever again."

"But . . . "

"Do you hear me?!" He shouted, as he did when he was afraid people weren't listening to him.

"But Dad . . . "

"I'm only telling you one more time before you're disowned," he said.

"Dad, they say you murdered their father. They almost killed me. I think I deserve to know what happened. I found the police report, too," my tone was now relentless.

He paused so that I could hear only his heaving breathing through the receiver. While my father was one of the toughest men you could possibly even make up and had endured more than three lifetimes' worth of struggle, he knew when he was cornered.

"If you want to know what happened, find the Yupik bear guide named Harry Frank. You are no longer welcome in our home in Hillsborough," he said, and once again hung up so that the receiver sounded as if it was thrown.

I called back three times. Each time he picked up the receiver and immediately hung up, so that my mother couldn't answer. I could hear my mother's voice the third time, elevated by an imploring tone. But my father's tyrannical side had emerged once again, on par with when he'd committed me to his prior poverty, after I graduated from Stanford. The rug pulled at the last moment to join the Troy Shipping Company, leaving me jobless and virtually homeless.

The only difference was that now his actions could no longer hurt me. Somehow that moment I felt that I was my own man more than ever before. Though the loss of my hero in spite of everything, the man who'd come to America and lived the promised dream, had only just begun to sting. And the stinging would only deepen as I realized that I truly had no home which to return once again.

TWENTY

MY NEWFOUND CONFIDENCE AND CONFUSION QUICKLY gave way to an agonizing pain that I first attempted to cure with spending money and food. And spending money on food. And alcohol. I would break my promise to my mother. I went down to the restaurant on the first floor of the Captain Cook, it's dimly lit open-air atmosphere perfect for the agony I felt to be on display. I had the last one hundred dollars from my per diem, that would be renewed in three days, and intended to spend it all on whatever manner of irresponsibility I could.

"A shot of whiskey and a beer," I said to the waiter, whose eyebrows raised at my double order. When he returned I said, "Bring me another beer after this. I'll be ready by the time you get back." To which he politely complied. I had a good buzz going by the time he brought the second beer, having washed the shot of whiskey down with the sweet taste of barley. "Bring me some bread. I'm having the halibut," I said, already tipsy. "And I want another beer." This line of terrible interrogation lasted until I'd consumed my fifth beer, and with the perfectly baked halibut and potatoes churning my stomach, as well as half a loaf of rich bread and butter, I was ready to get drunk on Fourth Street.

The intense sadness I was feeling was sufficiently numbed, and the thought that kept running through my soused consciousness was that my entire life—or what I could remember of it, had been a lie. Stolen. And by the trigger of my father's rifle. His "misfire" had ensured he would end up with the millions of dollars he had and was still enjoying. And placed two children within the orphanage—one was now an impoverished bear-hunting guide, and the other a woman of the night. They had no one to fend for them, to create a trust.

I stumbled under yellow-orange streetlights in intensifying rain, so that I could see the drops I felt, headed for Balto's, a favorite Anchorage watering hole, for my "Fourth Street vacation". This was the derogatory term my father had given to the behavior he said he witnessed from his clients, who when returning from the wilderness to the city, from hunts and other journeys, routinely went on what we would call a "bender" in California. Three or four days of uninterrupted drinking. I was returning from the wilderness of my misconceptions and misbeliefs. About my father. About myself.

And I still had no clue what I would do about it. Lost. Newly homeless.

"Grand Marnier," I said to the bartender, an Athabaskan man with long hair and an unassuming facial expression. "Make it a double."

As he slid the drink down the bar, he said, "What? Did she leave you?" It was clear what I was there to do.

"Worse," I said, performing my best impersonation of my sober self.

A chubby but not burly man with long, gray hair sat down next to me.

"How do you know what you know? Why is there something and not nothing?" He said jovially. Again with the fast Alaska friends.

Taking a long sip, allowing the orange liqueur to burn the back of my throat, I said, "I don't know anything, and there's something because of a cruel joke."

He smiled. "Sounds like you've either had too much or not enough," his jovial tone tempered by my nihilism.

"Both," I said, allowing the burn to spread to my stomach and torso. I only drank Grand Marnier when I wanted to achieve the same repose I'd enjoyed for the better part of two weeks after my accident on the ocean. Only now with an end in sight if I do transfer to UCSF.

"Well, the weather's the same as San Francisco," he said, more jovial. "At least it's not too much or not enough."

"What are you doing here?" I asked.

"I'm here to see the Northern Lights," he lent, believably. "If these damned clouds would just lift."

"Well, you want to be in Fairbanks this time of year for them. At least that far North," I offered. I felt the alcohol, which had begun its work at dinner at The Captain Cook, was beginning to serve its purpose. I could barely feel the unacceptable feelings I had after the phone call with my father. I knew my judgment would soon be lacking. And the feelings would be buried somewhere deep inside of me, a puppeteer dangling strings on my heart and actions.

"That's where I'm headed tomorrow," he said, sounding even more distant.

Why is there something and not nothing? How do I know what I know? I repeated to myself. I felt a sudden rush of sadness followed by anger, realizing the alcohol was in heated battle with my emotions.

"Another," I called over to the bar tender. "Whatever you do when you're there, don't ask for Vladimir and Natalya Bugaev," I said, unaware of what a ridiculous proposition this was, how porous my perceptions had become.

"Why do you say that?"

"My father killed their father," and at these words his jovial nature ceased. It was clear that he had come to Alaska to have a good time, and my state was now a great destroyer of affability.

"I'm sorry to hear that," he said. "That must be a lot for you to deal with. If you'll allow me to introduce myself more formally, I'm Rich Dawson. I'm a clinical psychologist."

"Aren't we all?" I said, still cynical.

"Now isn't the right time for you, but if what you're telling me is the truth, then I'd recommend you talk to someone about it."

"I can't afford that shit," I said, my words beginning to slur after another deep sip of Grand Marnier.

"Believe it or not, what you're doing can be healthy, though you can only escape for so long. Talk to someone," were the last words I remember him saying, before I began to time-travel.

How do you know what you know? Why is there something and not nothing?

I stayed at Balto's until the bartender cut me off, and judging from my previous experiences with Grand Marnier, it probably didn't take much longer. I don't really remember. My memory of the remainder of the night appears fragmented, most vividly of Rich Dawson and his advice, but then it seems at one point I was shoveling popcorn into my mouth at the bar next door, doused with Tabasco sauce, and then returning for a Balto burger, which was a mix of beef and reindeer meat, topped with fried halibut; at one point at a different bar I was encouraging a woman to dance with me after playing Led Zeppelin's "When the Levee Breaks" on the juke-box, my irresponsibility building, I remember the angry face of a native man outside as I accosted him for cigarettes, having spent my hundred dollars down to the point I didn't think I could afford my own pack, I remember standing, staring at the yellow-orange streetlights with my cigarette and imagining they were light portals to the afterlife, thinking "why not go there eventually—what could be the harm?"—and my final intimations of the night are swayed by feelings that I had finally blacked out, wandering from seedy establishment to seedy establishment, moments gracing the underbelly of Anchorage, their dark corners and the dark corners of my consciousness aligned, a hall filled with smoke and mirrors, I remember only the three-dimensional figure of a woman sitting on my lap, stealing my wallet with her hand where I wanted it, asking her, "Do you know Harry Frank!?"—the levee finally broken and gushing the river onto naive terrain, mumbling to myself, shouting at strangers as I stumbled through the spitting rain, "Do you know Harry Frank?!"—"Do you know Harry Frank?!?"—"The muffin man! The muffin man!"—laughing out loud— "Do you know Harry Frank?!? Why is there something and not nothing?!" And their faces of horror at the sight of my fully transmogrified condition, a zombie with alacrity, the past and future battling on opposite sides of a monstrous present, which had taken hold of me like the hungry jaws of natural justice.

When I awoke the following morning my head was pounding, my eyes burning, and I guzzled as much water from my hotel room faucet as I could. My wallet was gone. My ID, my last remaining dollars. I was now broke. In every sense. My head pounded until mid-morning, as I lay on bed, still dehydrated despite the water I'd consumed. But I had exorcised demons. The night of drinking was a temporary spiritual surgery for my anxiety at what I'd discovered—wound-inflicting but curative. I felt as though I'd smoked marijuana though I had no proof.

I recounted the final events of the night, tracing back to what Rich Dawson had suggested, knowing that he was right. I would seek counseling. Therapy. Whatever it's called these days. But I would go. I needed to go. I'd been through enough after what happened when I graduated Stanford, enough psychoanalysis and therapy to know that there were, indeed, the jaws of natural justice lurking beneath what I saw with my eyes, sensed with my ears, tasted with and spoke with my tongue. I needed help to process, to unite my consciousness in a way that was acceptable, so that I could keep going.

By lunchtime, I found that I could get out of bed. Go down to the Captain Cook's restaurant, where I could charge a meal to my room. If only Bob Fluor, the CEO who'd put me up there, knew that he'd failed. That I'd ended up on my Fourth Street vacation despite his generosity, that I'd failed him like I was made to feel I'd failed in so many other regards. I had been lied to and was now being honest with myself for the first time in a long while. Honest and compassionate. Tending to wounds. After the truth. An enemy of delusion.

And psychotherapy in the future and the present oozing of the broken yoke of an egg on my hashed potatoes with ketchup, followed by biscuits and gravy and pancakes with maple syrup, washed down with rich coffee and more water, would heal me. I gazed around the restaurant, its tables spread out and thin with customers at 11 a.m., as I ate the last of my breakfast. Broke. Gazing into the art gallery at the hotel at a sailing ship made out of baleen, from the inside of the mouth of a humpback whale, I resolved at that moment to journey to the center of my consciousness, like going to the center of the Earth. Drilling much further than we ever would in the North Slope. To illuminate the black hole I was mentioning. I'll invite whomever will listen to come on part of this journey, as I imagine it could end soon. Right here in this hospital room.

Sitting at my table, however, that following morning, after the bombs were dropped and the ground razed, reflexively I reached into the pocket of my still-damp jeans to produce my stolen wallet when the bill came. Instead, I found a crumpled piece of paper. In scrawled handwriting, black ink shocking my bleary eyes once more into complete clarity, it read:

HARRY FRANK 423-2756

Maybe the woman who'd stolen my wallet had given me an opportunity at revelation. If it was her and not someone else, they'd never know how gladly I would've traded my wallet for the piece of paper they'd left. How much more valuable this chance was. Though I'd never know from whom and on account of what that opportunity came.

TWENTY-ONE

"YOU WHO SUFFER NOW SUFFER MOST IN YOUR MIND," Ted's ghostly figure, diaphanous against the faded red-black says, his laser blue eyes beaming reason.

A tech stands in my room, taking an x-ray of my chest. I hear several additional sets of footsteps enter. It seems as though it's about time, as the regularity of my routine churns like clockwork.

"Coraline filed suit," Dominic Reagan says ominously. "Glower is a traitor, keeping us in limbo as he did until she could. Go get him," he orders the tech, whom he's never met.

"I'm only the—"

"—You heard me!" he shouts.

"It'd be a shame if something bad happened to Glower, like he fell out of this hospital window," Regina says, her voice dark as night. "If he lost a finger as my father lost his toes."

"Or if some acid were thrown in his eyes," Genevieve says, and I hear her produce a bottle from the cabinet to my left.

"Leave him to me," Dumb Dom says. "Ed, keep Genevieve company. And tell us where you're going, as we'll follow you."

A cellphone rings.

"Yes, Ozzie," Genevieve says. "What? They're what?! Sending him to UCSF? That's absurd. This is Glower's doing. We're ready to pull the plug on the bastard."

"Just get out of here, get Glower," Dom says. I hear Genevieve leave with Ed and Ozzie still on the phone. The tech leaves with the x-ray machine. "This is about to get out of control," Dom says to himself, alone with me.

The shoes clop into the room.

"Well-well-well, look who we have here," Dom says. "Is it Glower?"

"You ungrateful bastard," Regina says.

"Call the police," Dom says.

"What the hell are you talking about?" Glower says. "You're on my turf. You can't—"

"—You're a traitor," Regina continues. "We wanted the tube pulled, you saw his seizure, and now you're transferring him away from us, you're colluding with Coraline!" her voice's darkness intensifies. I hear her slap Glower's face.

"I am your host here, you crazy—" Glower says, wiping away what she's done.

"—Show us her e-mails," Dom says.

"Don't lie. We know the truth," Regina warns.

"And who told you he could be transferred to UCSF?"

"I made a clinical decision," Glower says. "Based on what's best for the patient."

"That's smart," Dom says.

"And a lie," Regina adds.

"Where are you sending him exactly?" Dom asks.

"To the eleventh floor. The Dover Neuro ICU, at the Parnassus campus."

"And why is that?" Dom says.

"Why?" Regina adds. "Why to UCSF?"

"Because I'm not going to be the one to pull the plug on him. There's new technology over there, and his advanced directive states that he wants everything done. I'm not going to let you and Genevieve commit him to death prematurely if we have these wishes written down.

I saw him look at me yesterday. He might have had a seizure. There's still a chance of a meaningful recovery, and we're sending him to UCSF for an experimental treatment, which might wake him up for good."

"Look at me straight," Dom says.

And I hear him produce the acid and Glower's horror as it enters his eye.

"My eye! My eye!" I hear Glower cry.

"You abusive bastard," the tech says, attacking Dumb Dom.

"My arm! You knocked it out of the skin!" he cries. "Here, Regina," he hands her the acid with his good arm, and Regina runs at Glower.

"What do you see now, good Doctor?" Dom says.

"Oh, oh!" Glower's cries are visceral. "I'm blind! Ed! Where is Ed?!"

"He's the one who told us about your treachery, your treasonous traitorous intentions. We are my father's family, we make the decisions—*not* you!" Regina shouts. Somehow we remain alone, without a commotion outside.

"Then Ted was innocent, my medical student son," Glower says in agony.

"Sniff your way from here, doctor," Regina says. "You're going to UCSF, too," she hisses, a snake. "You're going to experience what torture you've committed my father to. And if you tell anyone what we've done to you, we'll kill you. That goes for you, too," she snarls at the tech.

"My arm is broken badly," Dom says. "We need to get out of here."

I hear their two sets of feet leave and then Glower calling the nurses' station.

"I've had an accident," Glower says, as a collection of nurses begins to form outside. "I need the wash-out station."

"What monsters!" the tech says under his breath, before Glower's voice disappears behind the ICU doors, followed by a throng of horrified supporters.

TWENTY-TWO

I'LL BE BRIEF ABOUT THIS FOR NOW, WITH MORE LATER. The day before I went to the courthouse for the records, I went to a psychologist as Rich Dawson had suggested. Her name was Kim, and I told her I needed to get to the center of my consciousness, whatever that meant, though I was convinced it meant something that she could help with.

First she told me I'd always been afraid because my first memory, period, as I told her after she asked was of a musk ox hide from an animal that my father had killed, and also that I couldn't play outside as a child without fear of bears. Then she shortly got me to the point of saying my father was aloof building up the business, and before I could even really remember anything he was gone a lot, and now after decades of them not speaking about it, she made me realize it was because he was charged with killing someone and had to be gone for the trial. Oh, and I had come to believe it was for money.

"Can you see why you might have slight anxiety issues?" She relaxed her perfect posture in her lowly lit, comfortable, therapeutic office occupying a green building within view of my room at the Captain Cook.

"I do," I said after about forty minutes of talking about this, and also about how my mother had suffered while raising me. "Except you're forgetting what came of all those years of not talking about it. And that was toughness."

"That's fake toughness," she shot me down. "You've always felt as though you were in a battle zone. Beneath everything. Are you going to reach out to that hunting guide? Who was there when it happened?" She asked, leading me forwards into the emotional terrain I'd tread next, after what felt like hours of being where I'd been before. As though we were on an emotional timeline.

"I'll tell you after what I find tomorrow. I'm going to need your help with that at our next appointment."

"Okay," she replied, placing her notepad on the end table next to the leather chair after an hour of gently questioning and listening to me, as I grew more and more maudlin, the deeper we went. "Do you feel closer to the center?" She asked, innocently.

"I do," I said.

"I want to help you get where you want to go. But I need you to trust me," she said with a tone that seemed to say she was going faster with a client than she normally would, because of the urgency and what I was about to potentially discover.

I nodded, apprehensive.

For a minute we didn't say anything before I got up to leave. I felt somehow enlightened, as I had when going through the same process after leaving Stanford. Also protected from whatever I would discover at the courthouse tomorrow.

In those moments the low lights of her office lamps cast shadows of statues and figures on the walls and ceiling.

TWENTY-THREE

"BETTER TO BE A GHOST THAN SOMEONE WHO BELIEVES in smoke and mirrors," Ted's lost apparition says, his eyes metallic blue and emanating liquid light. "A ghost owes nothing to anyone, and only people who believe in you have the power to see you. Poor Tom! How awful it must be to be Steven Levinson, whom everyone sees, but is as real as a red herring."

I exhale once again into my breathing machine. We are at UCSF. On Parnassus. On the eleventh floor. I am too exhausted to take issue with his words.

He's taken special interest in our new whereabouts, because his father, Dr. Glower, was brought with me to this new hospital. The bed next to me, as his eye issues are considered intensive and neurological. Just like mine.

Truth be told, I didn't mind St. Mary's so much, despite what happened there. With my daughters. With Ken and Ed and Ted, and Thomas Mariner and Elie and Lia. And my seizure. I still have fond memories. The nurses were delightful in their own right. Despite Ed's machinations.

The room at St. Mary's itself was also comfortable. Comfortably tempered and with a comfortable temperature. And temporary. The other resident physicians, like Ken, were constantly joking with each other. Showing rapport. Getting food for one another. I would go back to St. Mary's, if necessary.

But I have come to UCSF, the University of California-San Francisco, so that my brain might be brought back to life, brought to light. The life they want for it. Despite Glower's punishment, here next to me, blind. They've brought him because he knows my case and my care best and can still speak. Despite what Genevieve and Regina say, this is what Danny wanted for me. I sense again that Danny is okay, though my excitement that I may be awoken soon takes precedence. What will I see?

"My son, Ted," Glower says to me. For the first time someone speaks to me who knows that I am here. Locked in here. "My son, Ted, Steve, is a crazy, homeless person, after I dismissed him from medical school. I feel so guilty."

"And that may not be the worst I am," Ted's ghost says, directly into Glower's consciousness.

"Wait, what was that?" Glower says out loud. "Ted?"

Several moments pass and Ted remains silent. Poor mad Tom.

"Steve," Glower says, "—Steve I just heard Ted's voice in my mind. I know I'm hallucinating. I was not friends with him, and he said he may end up worse than a homeless beggar."

"Bless you, father," Ted, the ghost who says 'Poor Tom', says to Glower.

"There he is again!" Glower cries. "You've brought me to St. Mary's," he says to Ted, his son. "In times of plague the crazy lead the blind. There is acid in my brain."

"Bless your bleeding eyes and acid brain," Ted says. "We are at Parnassus. At UCSF."

"Will you lead me to Parnassus?" Glower says. "I'll give you what's left of my accounts if you take me to Parnassus."

"I'll take you to Parnassus," the ghost who says 'Poor Tom' says, his eyes electric blue, his body shifting smoke in wind. He can't bear to tell his father that he is the spirit of a homeless person on the streets of San Francisco.

"I'll be humbled by all the strokes in their ICU," Glower says. "And if you take me to the window, I'll tell you what you need to know about me."

The ghost who says 'Poor Tom' touches Glower's arm. "Here," he says. "We're at Parnassus. I'll take you to the window."

TWENTY-FOUR

I WAS APPROACHING THE SECOND WEEK BEFORE I needed to embark back towards Fairbanks. I had discovered an awful proposition regarding my father and been disowned for confronting him about it. Which confirmed the awfulness without revealing the truth. The truth Kim was helping me discern without the possibility of my father's input. The truth I was going to the courthouse to uncover.

The massive cement edifice stood in contrast to the Anchorage Daily News building and its modern windows. The building appeared in the style of art deco, with corrugated columns and two massive revolving gold doors. Carved in relief were Roman figures, a woman donning only a bedsheet and a man holding a bow, with a bear and a wolf below them. I think it was supposed to be a commentary on humanity's place as presiding over nature, or something about natural law.

Unlike the archives at the newspaper, I wouldn't be able to simply go to some room and scroll through old papers. I'd have to request the files which had been kept locked somewhere all these years, some twenty-three since the accident occurred. As I entered the revolving doors there was no doubt that I'd enter.

A young man standing at the information desk asked if I needed help. His eyes were deep blue, his glasses large and bubbled out at me as they used to be, and his face was thin with a strong jaw. I imagined he was some kind of clerk or law student.

"Okay, sir," he said, after I showed him my military-issue ID that I thankfully kept in my suitcase and told him the details of the case. The

ID had been the thing to convince him. "I'll be back in ten minutes with an answer on how long it's going to be."

As he disappeared into a set of doors down the wide hallway with large oaken doors which must have led to the courtrooms themselves, I imagined, I began to ask myself: would another possible mental derailment have been worth it just to forget anything related to what I'd discover? Simply take the privileged childhood I'd been subject to, first in Alaska and then in California? Not to care what it had been built on? Who it'd been built on? And who might have suffered as a consequence?

But as I sat feeling the cool air of the foyer, with its marble floors serving as natural air conditioning, feeling the anxious sweat on my forehead begin to frost though not form droplets as it had before, I again became resolute. To know the truth if only once seemed worth whatever price I might have to pay. And I knew from my previous two experiences with madness that if the train began to run too hot on the rails, I had the wherewithal first to slow it down, then to stop it. I would have Kim's help, and my own experiences as a veteran. Both in Vietnam, and of the ward.

Besides, I was deep enough into my consciousness, a layer deeper than anything that could be rendered on the surface. And I would keep going deeper, as if towards the center of the Earth. Beyond the roots and the crust and to the core, even if it meant reaching nothing but a spinning ball of magma. What I was hoping to discover about my father, the surface of his behavior, spoke little of what remained beneath for me.

"Steven," the young man who'd helped me said like a North Vietnamese soldier in ambush, as I sat with my head against my hands, thinking what I've just told you. I startled and reflexively reached for my pocket as though a pistol might be there waiting. "Steven, I have some good news for you."

"What?" I said, again cooling my nerves as I was able to with Lia that day in Marin, my first experience with that kind of anxiety declaring itself.

"They're making copies of everything we have right now. From the docket to the briefs and depositions to the ruling. Alaska Territorial Fishery Service vs. Levinson. It's supposedly a famous case around here."

I only smiled anxiously, again trying to cool myself down from being startled. He seemed to sense that I was nervous, and again I think he respected me because I was a veteran. One of the few who still did.

"Give us another thirty minutes or so and I'll have the documents here waiting for you."

To kill time and ease my nerves I took a walk under clouds scattered like spun wool that afternoon, towards the statue of Captain Cook facing the inlet which now bears his name, stopping to look at him and ask questions—of what he experienced on his three voyages around the world—before returning to the courthouse. The statue spoke to me. And in short order the young man handed me the file that would reveal a quarter century's worth of secrets.

TWENTY-FIVE

"HEY, OZZIE," GENEVIEVE SAYS INTO HER CELLPHONE, on speaker. Ed is with her, having come to see his father. Glower has been taken for a procedure to ensure his eye sockets don't become infected. "What did my husband tell you? Is the legislature in session? Yes. I'm here with Ed."

"I told him Coraline was coming to San Francisco with her army of lawyers," Ozzie says with thick breath, as though he's been walking quickly, "And he just kind of laughed it off."

"Then don't worry about convincing him," Genevieve says to Ed, who she wanted in her plot to convince her husband, the Governor, to take action in international court against Coraline. She thinks because Coraline disclosed the details to Ed and Ed is a nurse, that his words might carry more clout. "Go to Dominic instead. He's on the fifth floor with the bone of his arm coming out of the skin from what that tech did to him, room 5056. Take the idiot the thing he loves most," and hands him several thousand dollars cash, "And don't say much."

"Whatever you want," Ed says, leaving. "I'm with you to the death."

"It's going to take a woman to get this done," she says to what she believes an empty room. "To finally give you the death you deserve, Daddy."

Her phone rings again and she answers it on speaker, because she's alone.

"I will soon be worth my weight in gold," Genevieve says to her husband.

"You aren't worth the dust on my grandmother's armoire," the Governor says. Marco's anger is palpable. "You're a branch disconnected from a tree. You're going to be firewood soon, for what you've done."

"What you've heard is false," Genevieve says, of what Ozzie's told him of Coraline's intentions. "She can't—"

"Your behavior is disgusting," Marco continues. "What you've done to your loyal father. If it were my child I'd feed them to the lions. Did Dominic put you up to it? That moron with an IQ of 60? The same as the animals you're going to be fed to—"

"You're pitying an animal himself," Genevieve's words begin to cut at me. "Aren't you the Governor of New York? Do you think Coraline's pitiful lawyers have a chance against us? Because they're from France? I always knew you were a coward!"

"And you're a devil!"

"You vain fool!" She retorts.

"If you weren't a woman, I'd . . . " Marco stops himself.

Suddenly Ed re-enters the room.

"Dominic is dead," he says, clearly having run six flights of stairs. "He developed sepsis overnight . . . from the arm the tech broke . . . throwing the acid in my father's eyes . . . and died . . . just ten minutes ago. That was the code they just called overhead."

I see the horror on Genevieve's face.

"You threw acid in Dr. Glower's eyes?!" Marco's voice comes through the phone, shaking me to my core.

"A tech . . . tried to stop us . . . and broke Dominic's arm badly," Ed is able to get out.

"Poor Dr. Glower," Marco says with animus.

"I'm going . . . to meet Regina. She sent you an e-mail. You need . . . to answer it soon," Ed concludes, before leaving again.

"You're going to pay for what you've done, Genevieve," Marco says for the third time, this time with the most force. "One way or another I'll make sure of that."

She hangs up on him without saying a word, and with Ed gone it suddenly feels as if six people are missing in the silence of my room. Where only the sounds of my cuff, ventilator, and monitors' quartet continues.

"I will and I won't," Genevieve says. "And I hope Ed and I can meet each other soon. My sister is a widow now, and I know how quickly she falls in love. If I can only run away with Ed and leave my controlling husband—I don't care what office he holds—then it will be as if I've died and gone to . . . " Before she can complete her thought, something catches her attention in the hallway. And she's gone, too.

Could what's on the other side truly be that much worse than what I'm in, what I've been in, since the accident? It more or less begs the question: what is it about our minds, what rests so near the center of our consciousness, that we want to keep living all the time? It seems going from insanity to sanity is the goal of every adult life.

In a few minutes I hear what distracted Genevieve to leave, and it's a few of the same voices that have visited me before, with one new addition.

"Here, it's this room," Thomas Mariner says.

"He's been here a few days," Elie adds.

"They say it won't be long before they connect the device," Thomas says, willfully oblivious.

"And were you still planning on being here?" Ferris says, aggressively.

"Listen, Ferris," Thomas says. But then it's as if he didn't think of what he wanted to say, or his good nature got the better of him.

"I'm just kidding," Ferris backs down a little bit. He's merely testing Thomas, who he already knows to be too accommodating.

"You two need to cut it out," Elie says. "Before I send you back to London. You've been too drunk and high that past two nights to even function," she shows her class and defuses Ferris's insolence.

"I'll go wherever I want," Ferris says. "Maybe I'll go see Danny."

"They wouldn't let you join the Army if you paid them," Elie says.

"He's doing some kind of operation currently anyway," Ferris says. "Instead of door-to-door salesman, it's like door-to-door FBI."

"Like your fantasy," Elie says. "Thomas here is the only one in the room who's done any investigative work."

"If you only knew how much I've investigated the doctor whose theories made the technology they're going to use on Steve," Ferris says.

"You mean Gideon?" Elie asks, speaking towards Thomas.

"Can you both please shut up?" Thomas says, as if collecting his thoughts. "What really matters here is that we need to tell Danny that this is happening. He clearly doesn't seem interested in communicating with Carmelia, as when she's tried to tell him, he never responds. He'll have access to the satellite phone sometime next week. Who's going to tell him? Like, he should probably be here for it."

"I don't think they'll let him," Elie says.

"His father is a billionaire," Ferris says. "They'll let him."

"As if having money lets you tell the military what to do?"

"Let me handle it," Thomas says. "I've been talking with Lia. We can all tell him. They'll make an exception for a dying family member."

For a moment their plan is hatched. I feel a sudden rush of warmth knowing that I might see Danny soon. Somehow this is mixed with the sadness of my prior insanity, a cocktail of hope and sadness and madness and self-pity for what my daughters are doing. For what I've, by proxy, done.

I try to travel in time and to probe Danny's friends' spirits, but Ferris's is too weak and instead of Poor Tom's electric eyes, I'm only getting a puff of Ferris's stale cologne. Elie's seems too porcelain and delicate and I'm afraid if I come too close, I might knock her off a table and she'll shatter into a thousand pieces.

TWENTY-SIX

WITH MY RIGHT HAND CLENCHING THE FILE I LEFT THE courthouse that afternoon, feeling as if it were the first day of the rest of my life. I stopped for a large coffee at the coffee shop in the Captain Cook, before returning to my room, which I held only for another two days. Before I'd head north again to meet Ethan, my own personal fortune seemingly waiting in the wings. Despite my current poverty.

I sat down at the desk facing Susitna and began going through the papers. First was the docket which listed the trial with the name the clerk had given me, "Alaska Territorial Fishery Service vs. Levinson". I guess because Vladimir and Natalya were still children and apparently there was no mother present, and the accident had occurred on public land, it was the local authority who served as the prosecution. The charges of "involuntary manslaughter" were brought against my father. Which carried a maximum sentence of eight years, as well as fines.

To the local authority, it appeared the terms of the case were clear. At least it seemed that way by the end to the Judge, named Henry Spruce. But first, as the territory's brief, written by an attorney named Messina—my father's defense attorney was named Sedgwick—laid it out:

On the evening of May 26th, 1951, Herman Levinson and Dmitri Bugaev were engaged in a planned, guided bear hunt on the Dalton Highway on the Southern Brooks Range north of Fairbanks, Alaska. Their unlicensed guide's name was Harry Frank. At approximately 9 p.m. a mature male grizzly bear they had been stalking to harvest became hostile, approaching them at a rapid speed. Herman

Levinson discharged his weapon unnecessarily at close range in the direction of Dmitri Bugaev, who stood between him and the attacking bear. Mr. Bugaev was poised to fire and capable of defending himself. The discharged firearm led to Mr. Bugaev's death by bullet wound to the chest and lower neck. The bear escaped after being wounded.

Here it was, in stark terms. The details of what happened.

I wondered if the territory had used the "close range" language as proxy for the fact that my father had won the Alaska sharpshooting championships. Kind of an Elliott Ness thing. Also, how had the bear been wounded, I wondered? Had my father shot both Dmitri and the bear? No matter what scenario was true, it seemed the case had rested on my father's testimony and the testimony of their hunting guide, then thirty-four-year-old Athabaskan man, Harry Frank. In fact, it appeared both had been deposed and testified, though for some reason Harry Frank's testimony was missing from the files I'd been given.

My father's portion of the testimony contained the following exchanges:

Sedgwick: Mr. Levinson, please tell us about the evening of May 26th, 1951.

Levinson: My friend, Dmitri, and I were stalking a grizzly bear and it attacked us.

Sedgwick: And in what manner were you hunting the bear?

Levinson: With rifles. Dmitri had a bow, but he also had a pistol. I had a rifle.

Sedgwick: And in what manner did the bear attack you?

Levinson: We were approaching for Dmitri to attempt to get a shot with his bow. But we came too close.

Sedgwick: How close?

Levinson: Probably forty feet.

Sedgwick: And then what occurred?

Levinson: The bear heard Dmitri break a branch while crouching to shoot, became startled, and charged at us.

Sedgwick: And approximately what size was this bear? Height and weight?

Levinson: I'd estimate that when standing, probably over nine, maybe ten feet. Maybe twelve hundred pounds.

Sedgwick: And what action did you take to dispose of this ten-foot, twelve hundred pound bear?

Levinson: I discharged my firearm.

Sedgwick: No further questions, your Honor.

The prosecution then cross-examined my father, as follows:

Messina: Mr. Levinson, isn't it true that you discharged your firearm that night at an estimated distance of less than fifteen yards?

Levinson: Yes.

Messina: And Mr. Levinson, isn't it true that, based on your winning the state sharp-shooting championship the previous year, that you are capable of shooting a six inch target from up to three hundred yards?

Levinson: Yes.

Messina: And Mr. Levinson, isn't it true that your friend, Dmitri Bugaev, possessed a pistol and was aiming at the grizzly bear that was attacking you as you shot him?

Sedgwick: Objection, your Honor, speculation.

Hon. Spruce: Sustained.

Messina: As you shot in his direction?

Levinson: Yes, Dmitri had a pistol. But I didn't think…

Messina: And isn't it true, Mr. Levinson, that only two weeks prior to this event, the rail shipping company that you owned through partnership with Mr. Bugaev, The Troy Shipping Company, had been given a lucrative contract with the United States Air Force?

Sedgwick: Objection, your Honor, relevance.

Hon. Spruce: Overruled.

Messina: Mr. Levinson?

Hon. Spruce: Answer the question, Mr. Levinson.

Levinson: That is true, although—

Messina: No further questions, your Honor.

So my father had been required, before the judge and jury, to reveal the nature of the contract. The one that meant I got to grow up a resident of Hillsborough. I hadn't known it was for the Air Force, but it makes sense, as the United States was building a base near Fairbanks at the time, a response to the Japanese having briefly held several Aleutian Islands during the War. I hadn't known they'd signed the contract two weeks prior to the accident. I hadn't known the bear was ten feet tall and weighed over a ton.

Regardless of what I wasn't able to find in the papers, namely Harry Frank's testimony, I decided to jump ahead to what the jury had decided, which was contained in the judge's ruling. It read:

The defendant is found not guilty by the jury based on a lack of a preponderance of evidence that his firing his weapon, leading to the death of Dmitri Bugaev, constituted an unlawful but unintentional act. While Mr. Levinson is not convicted of the crime of involuntary manslaughter, he is neither completely exonerated. The guide, Mr. Harry Frank, was also unlicensed at the time of the hunt, which is a crime in the territory. Mr. Levinson is fined $10,000 which will be placed in a trust for the children of Dmitri Bugaev, and will be required to serve two-hundred hours of community service in the arena of firearm safety and wildlife preservation.

"A lack of preponderance of evidence"? Looking through the evidence file itself it seemed the judge's words rang true, as there were only a few minor reconstructions of the angle of the shooting and a few photographs of the spot where the accident occurred. The remainder of the authority's case could only rest on testimony. Still, why was Harry Frank's testimony missing from the file? It was this vicissitude that sealed my decision on whether or not to call the number I'd been left by the stranger who'd taken my wallet, while surviving my "Fourth Street Vacation". Though I was still dealing with the shame I felt from my behavior.

But first, I paused to take in the entirety of what I'd discovered. It was making sense why my father had been so aggressive with me on the phone. Our entire fortune had been built on his killing his business partner, the one who'd given us the opportunity to come to this country in the first place. He'd barely avoided jail time. And now I had the documentation to prove it.

I felt the need to call someone, though I didn't know whom. I thought I could call Ethan, though I knew I'd be telling him once I got to Fairbanks as it was. I could call Harry Frank, but decided instead to wait until the day before I left Anchorage. Instead I chose to call Kim and schedule an appointment for the following day, before I left Anchorage again. To channel the broken yoke and journey still further to whatever lay hidden in the depths of my still-frozen heart.

TWENTY-SEVEN

"WHY DID MR. SARKOZY RETURN TO FRANCE?" KEN ASKS the social worker. The social worker was asked to call Coraline, who is miraculously in San Francisco.

"Because he had some national matters to attend to," the social worker says.

"Did he leave anyone with Coraline? Who's in charge?"

"A marshal named Luc from the French government."

"What was her reaction to what I gave you to send to her?"

"She began crying when she read the part about Steve here, and I had to ask her to calm down when she read the parts about her sisters. What they'd done, both their intentions towards Steve. She also believes what happened to Dr. Glower may not have been an accident. Apparently, Dom has a history of threatening people with their lives after he does terrible things to them."

Ken pauses, and I hear the fear permeate his breath.

"Was this before her husband returned?"

"No, after." The social worker sounds more hopeful.

"Well, the good news is that Steve is still here," Ken says, sincerely. "I'm sure he's still there. Every time I mention Coraline or anything about the situation, his monitors go off. I'm not sure if that's good or bad."

"Maybe we should just have Coraline come by. When the others aren't around."

"I think you're right," Ken says, as his attention turns to two sets of footsteps entering my room. "Hi there," he says.

"Hello," Elie's voice emerges from the red-black, a liquid crystal.

"Hello," Ferris echoes.

"Here to see Steve?" Ken asks.

"We are," Elie returns.

"Where's . . . Thomas?"

"He's in dispose," Ferris says. "Had a little too much fun last night." Again, the sarcasm peppering Ferris's voice lets me know of his intentions.

"Well, is there something I can help you with?"

"We're trying to get an idea of when they're going to . . . " Elie trails off.

"When they're going to . . . " Ferris attempts to help, but then it's clear to me that they're trying to come up with the name of the procedure that's going to happen to me. To try to wake me up.

"The thalamic ultrasonic stimulator?" Ken suggests.

"Exactly," Elie says.

"The plan is early next week."

"This is Thursday," Ferris says. "Are we talking Monday?"

"We were hoping you could tell us. Aren't you trying to get in touch with Steve's son?"

"Right," Ferris says. "We're talking to him tonight or tomorrow."

"And is he planning on being here?"

"Right now, we don't know," Elie says. "There's a chance he'll fly in over the weekend."

"Let us know when you know for sure," Ken says. "We want to make sure, based on prior experience, that family are here. It's a pretty incredible moment if it works."

"We'll be sure," Ferris says, with a tincture of tone thinning his voice that lets Ken know he doesn't respect him.

"Thanks for asking," Elie says. "Glad we caught you at a good time."

"Sure. Just let somebody know as soon as you know," Ken says, before leaving.

For a moment I hear Elie whisper something to Ferris that I miss. And when I try to listen to Ferris he speaks at an inaudible level.

"If last night wasn't such a disaster," I hear Elie say out loud, as if purging her thoughts of it.

"I've never seen someone put back that much bourbon," Ferris says. "And was he really wearing sunglasses inside?"

"I think he's starting to understand," Elie says.

"Understand what?"

"What a mess all of this is. The easy thing for me to do would just be to break up with him. Except then he keeps talking about how I'm everything Anna wasn't. And then I start to feel guilty, because I know I'm not. That he's literally just grafting whatever he wanted Anna to be on to me, and that I'm really a terrible person. For doing this to him. Asking him to come out here."

"Well," Ferris says, thinking. "The easy thing for me to do, maybe the most compassionate thing, would be to kill him. I know a guy in North Beach who says he'll do it for free. Otherwise we send him back to Chicago or wherever, having lost his fiancé over the stuff we did with him. Did to him."

"I know," Elie said with a sympathetic lilt in her voice for Thomas. "The thing is," she tried to decide whose side to take in that instantaneous, intuitive way she did, "I could also anoint him."

"Oh please," Ferris says. "Like you're his savior now. He's like your play-toy. The flavor of the month. Shit, the week. Why don't I just kill him?"

"Ferris," Elie's voice sounds confused again. "Ferris you're a maniac."

"A maniac who's going to anoint Gideon's work and take a huge piece of the pie for myself. We anoint billionaires. Wait until next Monday. The press is going to be here. Danny is going to be here. And Thomas is going to be hiding somewhere, like back at your apartment."

"Whatever," her voice now sounds the furthest it could possibly be from caring about Ferris's financial games and business aspirations, and is fully human, fully empathetic. "I could just as easily have Danny kill you for what you've done."

Ferris is suddenly silent, completely stopped in his tracks by her words. He then laughs as if the possibility that he would ever die was equally absurd.

TWENTY-EIGHT

"I'M SORRY, STEVEN," SHE SAYS, WITHOUT PURSING HER lips, and with the most empathetic tone you could possibly even make up. Like my mother at times, though I fight the thought that Kim has anything to do with her. I'm not here to be loved. I'm here to set a few things straight that might be hidden from me. Deep down in there. At the center. "Can you tell me more about how you felt when you . . . confirmed what you'd suspected? Or maybe even better, can you tell me how this affected you, especially ways you didn't anticipate?"

"I don't know that I really felt anything," I said, kind of telling a half truth. "Why is that?"

"I have a few ideas," she said, and then made a face with open eyes and a slightly raised perfectly manicured brow as if also asking if I wanted to hear them. I nodded. "The first is that you were trained not to feel. Both from your family, but also from the military." I paused in agreement. "The second is that you were, maybe still are, in shock. Our emotional lives tend to shut down when presented with overwhelming information. Which this certainly qualifies. Which is why I need you to take a moment and tell me how you're feeling."

For a moment I closed my eyes and took a deep breath, which was acceptable to a therapist, I always thought. For another moment I tried to feel something, and then realizing said, "I feel as though I have an emotional callous for my father." She looked at me as if this was interesting. Instead of asking me to continue she just kind of wanted me to. So I did. "Or maybe like the dead skin is falling off."

"Good, Steven," she said. "Good. Let it fall off. How does that feel?"

"I guess kind of sensitive."

"Yes," Kim said as if we were getting somewhere. She waited again, repositioning her arm so that her chin rested on her first three knuckles. "Yes, continue."

"But it's not painful," I said, again going wherever I was being led.

"I think you're ready to start feeling some of your real emotions about this," she encouraged, half-smiling. "Good or bad. Don't be afraid." I paused. "What's the first emotion that's coming to you now, just say it, don't even think about it."

"Sad," I said, quickly realizing I wanted the noun and had instead chosen the adjective. Which is probably what she wanted anyway.

"I'm sorry," Kim said. "I'm sorry you're feeling sad. Sadness is usually the result of a feeling of loss. What do you think you've lost through all of this?" I knew she had her own ideas but for the first time in a long time as I allowed the sadness to descend into the well of my heart, seeping into my chest and enveloping all the way around my back, I also began to feel a tension lift as I had during our first session.

Rather than mince words, I just said, "My hero."

"Wow," Kim said. "Your hero. Your father was your hero?"

"Yes," I said, feeling a rising in my throat and a fullness glaze my eyes.

"Now, Steven," Kim said, after a long silence that led me to this comfortably uncomfortable place. "What else are you feeling?"

It seemed as though a switch had been turned inside of me. Whereas until I left Stanford I'd been the paragon of rationality, I also knew both from what I had gone through and from what Lia had offered to me without offering anything, that Rich Dawson had been correct. I needed to go places I otherwise wouldn't go on my own.

"Anger," I said, this time choosing the noun.

"Good," Kim said. "I'm sorry you're feeling anger. That's understandable. Anger is the result of injustice. And can actually be a productive emotion, if we don't let it consume us. Just like sadness. Anger is like fire. It can heat your house and cook your food; or burn it down if it's uncontrolled. Now let me ask you, Steven, you aren't thinking of acting on your anger, are you?"

"No."

"Good."

"But . . . " I said, unable to speak, the combination of the sadness she'd brought out and the anger momentarily limiting my language.

"It's important to acknowledge our anger, and use it as fuel. And whatever you do, Steven, *do not*," she said for the first time with such emphasis, " . . . do not internalize or deny it, because it's just as quickly a path towards your own emotional and spiritual destruction as uncontrolled sadness." She paused to allow my anger to pass, temper, or intensify, which it did in various forms before I returned to my prior calm. "I think what you're doing up here, trying to earn your independence from him, is possibly the most healthy thing you could be doing with your anger. It sounds like you knew it was there before, and now you're simply more conscious of it. I hope you are."

"I am," I said. "I'll use it as fuel."

"The fact that your father won't speak to you or see you has got to be fuel, and not an uncontrolled fire. What you discovered about his past, and therefore yours, needs to be a cause for peaceful reflection, rather than self-destruction. You've already had your 'Fourth Street Vacation' or whatever you called it. Now it's time to be compassionate with yourself—and someday, I hope, with him." These words she spoke as if delivered from a pulpit, and for a moment I felt as though I was embraced by a deeply spiritual presence. If she hadn't said anything else

I would have at least felt this. Then she continued. "Are there any other things you're feeling? How about fear? Are you afraid of anything?"

"Yes," I said. "I'm afraid of…" and I couldn't even really come up with what, though all these years later I realize it was that I'd never see or speak to him again. That this would die not only on his conscience and heart but also on mine. What in the past had been my raw processing power, that allowed me to reason my way through situations, was becoming a different kind of processing, the kind that ran on its own schedule, that you could try to rein in but was wild like a horse, that could carry you to great heights or submerge you to great depths, the kind you could only listen to, only speak by whispering to the thunder, and let invite you in—and you needed to go in to sit next to its electricity without judgment, to let this kind of truth be what it needed to be, rather than to force your formulas on it. "I'm afraid this will never be resolved."

"Steven," she said, as if having anticipated my response. "That's not up to you. So just let it go. Sometimes what happens in the past never dies for those it happens to; except for those who live in its shadow, like you've now discovered—you're living in its shadow—the best thing you can do is just find your own spark, that lights your own match, let it breathe, let it burn, then find a torch, and let it both guide you and warm you."

At that moment I decided I wanted to be with Lia. I knew she was the light Kim was referring to without Kim having to say it and without Lia having to know it, though I suspect she knew; though what I felt without seeing them as I had that day in Marin, were the same stars and celestial figures. It was probably the moment I decided to invite her on that hike in Marin. The one I'd give anything, even my life, to go back to, to relive that moment.

"Please promise me you'll light your own match against this darkness," Kim continued.

Sadness. Anger. Fear. By letting a little of each in, I journeyed beneath my thinking brain, still closer to the center, avoided them crashing through the door eventually, as they always did. More violently. Asking no permission.

It's something I'm trying to remember to do, or how to do, as I lay here in dispose at Parnassus, approaching what I believe to be the ultimate center of my consciousness, three days from my possible re-entry into the same world where the same grizzly acts take place. Where my daughters fight through their anger, sadness, and fear at what's going to happen to me. And to them when I'm gone. Clawing and gnashing and thrashing at each other and at me, at Dr. Glower, trying to escape a burning building. They're all showing their true colors, as I began to show then in my late twenties. Stress is the most honest of palettes.

TWENTY-NINE

THE MORNING ROUTINE IS DIFFERENT AT PARNASSUS, IN the Dover Neurological Intensive Care Unit at UCSF. I don't know if it's because they're preparing me to wake up, if Gideon's invention works, or if it's because I'm lying here, blind and mute, with a blind doctor as my only company. Who I can't speak to. Who speaks about me. With Ed now only an occasional visitor, to both his father and me, I feel as if an ominous presence has been lifted.

The smells of Parnassus are also different. I'm not sure much different, as most intensive care units seem to have the same sterile, musty aroma. Or anyway, I can't tell if it's just that I smell different. The breathing tube is less cumbersome, and I feel that my lungs have strengthened. They're even talking about letting me breathe on my own for the first time on Monday.

Somehow I feel Dr. Glower's presence more forcefully, as if his blindness, mirroring my own, has brought us into a metaphysical communion. Trapped, red-black companions in space. The same place I saw Ted, the ghost who said 'Poor Tom', except only he can see me there, while I remain unable to speak to him. With this knowledge, Glower directs my care. While receiving his own.

I hear footsteps enter my room. I assume it is Thomas, Elie, and Ferris. Perhaps Lia, who comes nearly every day. The routine at Parnassus is similar to St. Mary's. The vacuum to remove saliva. The respiratory technicians, as the one who inadvertently killed Dominic, come to check my settings. Make sure the tube is secure. All on schedule. And now I hear more footsteps.

And yet her voice sounds like a sunrise.

"He looks so peaceful. While I know his mind can't be," Coraline says to someone. She has arrived for the first time and I feel her presence like a cavalry. "I wish you could bring him back to me now, instead of on Monday. Without those witches here, if you'll pardon me for saying that. What's happened must have made him crazy. What exactly do you have here to make him awake, again?"

"We have a means," I hear the voice of my neurologist, a woman, Dr. Eugene, say. "An ultrasonic thalamic stimulator, which is a fancy name for a machine that's going to restore his consciousness. Surely you've heard by now," she pauses. "Sleep is good medicine for him. And until then treat it as if he can hear you."

I hear a cellphone ring. It is Coraline's.

"Your sisters' lawyers are here," a voice with a French accent says on speaker.

"I know," she says. "We were expecting them." I wonder if it is her international attorney from Paris. "Dad," she speaks to me for the first time directly, and something deep stirs within me, "that's why we're here. To protect your business. The President of France's brother, our friend, heard what I told him. You'd be so proud of what I found after you sent me away, as I'm proud of you for fighting to stay alive. I hope we hear and see him on Monday."

"There's a good chance you will," Dr. Eugene says.

"Thank you for what you're doing. Though I'm still a little jet-lagged and should get back to the house I'm staying at."

"I understand," Dr. Eugene says. "It's a big weekend coming up before Monday. If I'm not in the building, I'm always available by phone. Day or night. Until Monday."

"Thank you," Coraline says, and clutching my hand for a moment, she pauses, and I hear a quiet wince, before she leaves.

"Edward," Dr. Eugene says. "Are you awake?"

Glower remains silent, but I sense that he is awake and merely not wanting to comment on what he thinks is best for me at the moment. I wonder if it's because he's afraid of what Regina and Genevieve will do to him. I hear Dr. Eugene's footsteps go out of the room.

"I wanted it this way, Steven," Glower says after we're alone. "I asked to be in your room. If they're going to kill me, I'll die trying to save you."

While I can't thank him, I sense the sincerity of his words. And for the moment feel protected. Until the next set of two footsteps enter. By the warmth I'm feeling on my face and the bright shade of red-black, I figure it must be afternoon.

"Steve," Elie says. "Steve I just spoke with Danny."

"He's going to be here Monday," Thomas says, with a relieved tone soothing his voice, as if he's decided something.

"Do you think he really can hear us?" Elie says. "This feels a little funny."

"That's what his neurologist, told us," Thomas says. "To treat it as though he can hear us."

Elie doesn't say anything as if she's worried about what I heard, unaware that she has reason to be afraid.

"What are you going to tell Danny when he's here?" Thomas asks.

"Thomas," Elie says, with her tone transitioning from annoyed to compassionate. "I need to talk to you first. I guess here is as good a time or place as any."

"I'd say we need to talk before Danny gets here," Thomas says.

"Tommie," she says with sincere compassion softening her voice, "—I think it's time we start talking about our future together." And from the tone of her voice, I can tell Thomas must be concerned about whether or not this is another break-up talk. Or she means the opposite.

"What do you mean?" Thomas says. "Aren't we living our future together already?"

"I mean," Elie says, "I've been doing some thinking. And wanted to tell you that, if you asked me to marry you, I would."

Thomas, ever the calm and collected one, does not immediately respond.

"That is something we should talk about," Thomas says after a moment, his tone both agreeing with her and keeping his distance. It's as if he's protecting himself from the headlong throwing of himself that he did with Anna, while wanting to keep the lifeline open that brought him to San Francisco.

"I mean," Elie's tone now sounds even more sincere, making me wonder if something happened with Ferris that's sealed her refusal of him. "After Danny couldn't ask me, even before he went off to Afghanistan, and after having you here even just for this past month, I think I'm finally happy."

"That's good to hear," Thomas's tone is colder. I still hear the hopeful softness beneath his doubts. "Are you happy?"

"I am."

"Good," he says.

"But I need to ask you something," Elie says as Thomas pauses to prepare.

"What?"

"Do you want to get out of town this weekend?"

The concrete and practical nature of her question catches Thomas off guard. As if she just asked for a cigarette.

"Ah, sure," Thomas says. "Where?"

"Let's go up to a place in Marin County called The Pelican. It's a nice English style hotel, and has a nice pub and restaurant. I feel like with Danny coming and Ferris, and what's happening on Monday, it might be the last chance we have to be together before a lot changes. There's another place I want to take you up there called McClure's Beach. We can hike down and have a bottle of wine in a cave."

"Sounds very nice," Thomas's convinces himself, belying his passion for her.

THIRTY

LEAVING ANCHORAGE FOR FAIRBANKS WAS ONE OF THE more difficult and liberating things I think I've ever done. It reminded me of leaving Vietnam, the discovery I'd made about my father almost like the war I had to fight within myself. Stretching into the distant past. And similarly, when I left Vietnam we hadn't won the war, as I hadn't won the war that was wrought by that past.

My heart prepared to fight or to run again as I viewed these billowing and slow-creeping clouds, moving as a slow-motion, inverted river, obscuring the mountains as the train overcame its inertia and we departed. I guess what my body and senses had learned in Vietnam were there to protect me, and while it wasn't full-alert-crisis like with Lia that day atop Marin, I could feel my heart begin to beat and I took a few deep breaths.

I hadn't called Harry Frank that morning as I'd planned, figuring I could put it off until the next day. I don't know why. I had called Ethan and he told me where to meet him, the address where we would disembark, just the two of us with a few other Fluor employees. To figure a way for the pipeline just east and then south of Fairbanks. Making its final descent towards Valdez. We were also supposed to talk about finances for our first two rigs, as well as plans to fly to Barrow the following spring when the pipeline would be completed.

As the train rolled away from Anchorage and we made our way towards Palmer, where the state fair was happening, I felt the layers of my anxiety begin to evaporate slightly. Like after solving a complicated math problem; that moment of relief when you've arrived at an answer. It wasn't a complete resolution or clear one, and so the feeling was more a residue of clarity. Deeper currents still churning.

My train arrived in Fairbanks that night after twelve hours north through inhospitable country. The whole time I kept thinking just how crazy and ridiculous it was that humans were even capable of building a means to transport a river of black gold across such terrain. I see it all so clearly from my spot at Parnassus now, the Dover Neurological ICU, a similar structure that I can hardly believe possible.

"Even Steven," Ethan said at the doorway to the house Fluor was renting on the northeast outskirts of Fairbanks.

"I'm about to get even," I said, smiling, happy to see my childhood friend.

Ethan and I had met first as neighbors—if you can call living a mile away a neighbor—as they were the closest family to us south of Anchorage. His family lived in a log cabin without running water and we used to play and swing on the rope in his yard in the summer time. Then we became school-mates at Eisenhower Elementary School until the fifth grade, when my father moved us to Hillsborough. He'd grown to be about my height, not tall but not short, and in his prime was muscular with wavy brown hair, brown, deep-set eyes, high forehead. The most compelling aspect of his appearances was a charismatic, almost maniacal smile.

Ethan's father, Brad Helms, was a former marine and had participated during the D-Day invasion on Utah Beach, the day after they landed. I think Ethan also helped me after Vietnam because I was a veteran and he felt guilty for taking a medical deferment for a heart condition he later told me was mostly made up, where there was a communication between two chambers that basically didn't cause him any symptoms. But it was diagnosed and his mother made him use it to avoid going where I went, where Camille, Red, and I ran through that field.

"Here, meet Nali," Ethan said, as a large, what looked like could only be a sled dog, approached me, rising on its haunches, standing so tall as to lick my face.

"Hey, Nali!!" I said. "Cut it out . . . haha . . . are you a good girl?" I petted her as she dropped to all fours. "She's beautiful," I said. "What is she?"

"You're not going to believe this, though you might," he said. "She's actually half wolf, half husky. Do you remember?"

Suddenly I was taken back in time twenty years, to when we were seven or eight. We used to play throughout his large backyard, which was dense with raspberry bushes that we used to pick and eat from, as well as the same thin conifers that grew on permafrost. One morning we were out there pretending to hunt a moose. With a deep growl we were approached by a snarling animal that looked very much like Nali. It stood there about fifty feet away, showing its teeth in waves of indignation. For a moment we were petrified the way children are by threatening animals. I'll never forget how my back tightened.

"Do you remember how we ran?" Ethan said, referring to how we'd turned from this wolf-dog and run what seemed miles, though was probably only a couple hundred yards, as the animal pursued us. At one point I fell and as I remembered this I remembered falling and spraining my ankle while Vlad chased me, triggering the heartbeat again.

When we got back to Ethan's house after Ethan fought the wolf off with a stick and we told his father, Brad was furious that the next neighbor over, who owned an animal who was half-wolf, half-malamute, had allowed it off his property. Without supervision. The neighbor said the animal got away on its own and was trying to return to the wild on its own; that it'd been trying to escape, and that doubly it had only chased us out of the instinct they have to chase smaller animals.

"I remember," I said. "Where'd you find her?" It had been almost a year since I'd seen Ethan as we'd both been out surveying with separate groups.

"Long story," he said. "But suffice to say she was half-wild when I found her. She's pretty well domesticated now. Won't ever eat unless I'm around."

The vagueness of his answer led me to believe he'd found Nali while surveying.

"Is she joining us?"

"Oh hell yes," he said. "How the hell are you, though?"

For a moment I was simply reminded of how much I enjoyed Ethan's company. He was warm and a bit crazy and everything you'd expect from someone who'd never left Alaska.

"I'm doing okay," I said. "But I've got news about my old man. Is there any chance we can leave the day after tomorrow?"

"For you, anything," he said, smiling. "But I have no idea what that means."

As Brad Helms had gone on to befriend Bob Fluor, the CEO of our company, on account of their military backgrounds, Ethan had enjoyed a kind of favored status in the company. This simultaneously fueled his carelessness and also made him serious during the hours he was working. Not wanting to disappoint his hard-ass father.

I went on to tell Ethan what I'd discovered about mine over a neat glass of scotch. Ethan had gotten out his black bear headdress, which he set on the table.

"No offense, but this is absolutely fucking crazy," he said, looking through the files I'd brought. Ethan had a way of saying difficult things soulfully so that it took the edge off. He knew my father more as a child knows other children's fathers, as we'd seen little of Ethan in California and before I reached out to him after I was honorably discharged from the Marines. "All I remember is that he never wanted to talk about Troy. Like the thing that was making him millions of dollars was a nuisance."

"I know," I said. "I had the same feeling my whole life. Except it's starting to make sense."

"So, do you think he did it?"

"I know he 'did it'," I said. "If you mean firing the shot. The question is, was it intentional? And I think this Harry Frank guy is the only one who might possibly know for sure."

"Because he was there."

"Because he was there."

"Well, you'd better call him. Hell, call him before you have too many of these," he said, picking up his glass before refilling it.

And believe it or not I think it was the scotch that finally gave me the courage and the wherewithal to call Harry Frank. I picked up the phone. 423-2756 shunked around the rotary dial. The phone rang and rang as it did in those days before everyone had an answering machine.

"This is bullshit," I said. "He's not even home."

"Who gave you that number?" Ethan asked.

"I don't . . . never mind," I said quickly, redialing, hoping I'd only missed a hole in the rotary.

The phone rang and rang again and I was feeling that sinking feeling take my stomach for a second time. As though I'd never reach a final answer. I felt stupid for waiting until now, in front of Ethan, too, for some reason. Like why hadn't I just called from Anchorage the previous day? And then I felt the full weight of my Fourth Street Vacation, having my wallet stolen and replaced with what was probably a fake number meant to give me the impression it was being put in my pocket, when all they wanted was my wallet. Which I hadn't even replaced.

I went to replace the receiver, acknowledging final defeat. But then I heard a voice come through the headset, faint and accented and a little confused.

"Hell-o," he said, with an uptick emphasis on the "O".

THIRTY-ONE

"17201 MARIJANE DRIVE," HE SAID, AFTER HANGING UP on me twice when I told him who I was, and the nature of why I was calling. Finally telling me the address where we'd meet the following day—remember, this was the 1970s. Because I wanted to see him in person.

Ethan let me drive his car and I left him and Nali at his cabin, traveling towards the opposite side of Fairbanks from where Vlad had almost killed me on account of whatever I was about to discover. For a second I was afraid I might pass Vlad on the street and he'd recognize and shoot at me again. I'd been shot at enough recently. The sky remained gray with the same drizzle as always permeated Anchorage, except the drops were a little smaller this far inland. More like a mist.

I weaved my way back through the woods where Harry had directed me. There stood a modest cabin with wood of the color it is, that is a little lighter, when a cabin is newer. The gravel ground beneath my feet and I kicked a little behind me, as the new stairs did not make a sound under my feet. I heard each footstep before opening the outer screen door and knocking on the inner, wooden one.

No answer.

I checked the address on the side panel of the door, which was correct. It was about nine in the morning and I realized we he hadn't said a definite time, just in "the morning." I carried the file they'd given me at the courthouse under my right arm. I began feeling stupid again, like why couldn't I have said a time? Now I might be waiting hours.

"Hey, Steven?" A voice suddenly emerged from behind me, and I spun around reflexively as if I had heard a gunshot in a Vietnamese jungle. Walking from the side of the long driveway and onto the gravel was a short, thin, strong and diminutive native man who appeared in his mid-60s, with a winsome smile. "Are you Steven Levinson?"

"Yes," I said, feeling the tension clenching my back relieved. I wondered if I'd ever felt this relaxed. "Harry?"

"That's me," he said, coming up the stairs. "I've been chopping wood."

He led me inside after shaking my hand and smiling again without saying anything. I wondered if he was as nervous as I was underneath everything. Or if he felt the same relief I had at seeing me. I imagined probably not. If anything, I gathered he was doing this only as an obligation to me. While he was friendly.

"Is this where you've been living?" I asked, not really knowing what I meant.

"I just moved here," he said. "Last year." The cabin was open on the inside just like Vlad and Natalya's, except we didn't need the low lamps for lighting. The light that came through the windows on all sides of the shared kitchen-living room was gray. "You drink coffee?" He asked.

"Yes," I said, taking a deep breath.

Sometimes what happens in the past never dies for those it happens to . . . Kim's words ran through my head again, as I tried to remember how to conduct myself.

"Sit down," he said, pointing to his "dining room" table, which was just kind of sitting in a space next to the kitchen and living room. The decor was sparse, most of the walls uncovered. He poured the coffee that was already made, and brought me a cup and sat down in the chair next to the kitchen while my back was facing the living room.

"Thank you," I said, taking the first sip, which always produced joy.

"So, you came here to learn about your father?"

"Yes," I said, surprised at how quickly he'd simplified the reason for my being there. His hair I now noticed was long and pulled to a ponytail behind him. He wore the large-framed glasses common at that time.

"Well, what do you know?"

I had placed the file on the table and reached for it as he asked. "Everything in here," I said, showing him the papers that included the testimony, the few pictures and other evidence the state had collected.

"I remember," he said. "You don't have to show me. So you went to the courthouse."

"Yes," I said.

"I guess it was inevitable," he said, taking a sip of his coffee and combing his hands over a few pages of the papers, as if reminding himself by touching them.

"Why isn't your testimony there?" I asked.

"Wait, it isn't?" he said, now thumbing through a few more pages.

"No," I said. "I figured it was the most important."

"I bet somebody stole it," he said, not giving a reason.

"Well, what did you say?" I pressed.

"It doesn't matter," he said. "The case is closed."

"But what did you say? Or, what can you tell me about what happened that night?"

He looked past me and out of the front window, as if recollecting. I didn't know if he was annoyed and ignoring the question. Then the expression on his face turned from kind and jovial and morose, almost wistful. "That was twenty-five years ago," he said rhetorically.

I paused, not wanting to disturb whatever thoughts were forming. For perhaps the first time, and in a very timely manner, against my will, I felt able to accept whatever it was that he was going to tell me.

"It seems to me like a dream now," he said. "I can't tell you exactly what happened."

"Was the bear charging?"

"When your father shot, yes," he said. "We'd been stalking it. Got too close. I think the same bullets that killed Dmitri wounded the bear. It happened faster than my fist," he lightly pounded the table.

He paused, silent for a moment, seeming first to struggle with, then find calm in what to say next.

"Did I think your father was a good guy? Yes. Did he have a lot to gain? Yes. Do I think he did it on purpose?" he paused. "I don't know. No one knows but him. I'm sorry. Sometimes we don't know why people do things. And maybe they don't either."

I waited a moment to see if he'd say anything more. Suddenly a rush of sadness came over me for what he'd had to live with, that I was only beginning to live with.

"So, do you know Vladimir and…"

"I know them," Harry said. "I trained Vladimir. He wanted to be a guide his whole life, since he was fifteen. He always thought the bear killed his father. I told him the bear did it."

"Then why did he want to kill me?" I asked. "Meeting him is what led me to you."

"He had a way of finding out," Harry said, again cryptically. "He just found out. The truth always comes out in the end. There's no hiding."

His words sounded as solid as Mount Denali. I could not tell if they were majestic or ominous.

"Vladimir spent a good portion of his life trying to kill the bear he thought killed his father?" I asked.

"Yes," he took another sip of coffee. "I let him. Until he just found out."

"That explains his reaction to meeting me," I said. I then quickly chose whether or not to try to see Vladimir and Natalya again, through Harry. "If you see them," I said, "tell them I'm sorry. Do you know Kira?"

"I know Kira," he said.

"Tell them I'm sorry," I said again, feeling all the guilt and anguish and remorse and pain resurfacing. "Thank you for letting me come here, for speaking to me," I said. "I think I'd better be going."

"First let me show you something," Harry said, sensing what I was feeling. It seemed he'd prepared something to show me.

I didn't say anything.

He walked slowly with a slight limp over to a bookshelf by the living room, selected a book and brought it over.

"This is a book written by my great-great-grandfather," he said. I took the book in my hands and read the back cover. It detailed that Harry's ancestor had been a chief amongst the Haida people, in what we now called the Queen Charlotte Islands. "He wrote every day in his journal for fifty years," Harry said. I was still having difficulty understanding why he was showing this to me.

"That's very interesting," I said. I'd never kept a journal or written anything. "You must be very proud."

"Last night after you called, I started thinking," Harry said. "I started thinking about the last twenty-five years. I must have written to my own journal a hundred times about that night. What I saw. The look on Dmitri's face after it happened, how the life left his body."

He looked at me now, instead of out of the front window. His expression was kind.

"My grandfather also wrote about the bad things that happened in his life. They took his journals and they're now in London. My wife, who died two years ago, before I moved here, and I went there, and I have a copy of many of his journals."

I again said nothing, realizing I had nothing to say to this.

"Steven," he said. "When I started thinking about what to tell you, I thought of my grandfather. How he kept living and kept writing in spite of everything. The way of the Haida continues to this day, one hundred and fifty years later. You will be fine," he said. "Keep going. Keep fighting."

The rush of sadness and anguish and even anger subsided at his words, though I could only approximate their meaning. But my intuition knew what he was saying. That history is littered with grave injustice. I felt a resolution at his words. Not that I should, but that I would do something. I suppose it was from that moment I decided to start my fishing business in the Queen Charlotte Islands. Or what's now called 'Haida Gwai'. To be nearer Harry Frank and his ancestors. And to give something back to them.

"Thank you," I said to Harry, and I knew he understood everything else from the way I had conducted myself. From what was unspoken and the very fact that I was there.

"Thank you," he said.

I collected the files on the table, shook his hand without words, and departed.

The joy and exaltation I was expecting for a clear answer was equal to anything I'd felt before to that point in my life—save what Camille and I had shared for that week near Cao Lanh. Something solid. Based in a pursuit of truth. Whereas Camille and I had been engaged in the beautiful fallacies lovers fall into when the world is collapsing around them. Like Thomas and Elie now. I was trying to build a world then. And that world would ultimately remain incomplete.

Ethan and I celebrated, nonetheless, that I had some answer, that I'd come this far, even to a destination as gray as the sky in Fairbanks. We celebrated for the remainder of the night, at times growing jovial, him telling wild and hilarious stories, at times donning the black bear headdress, and then reflecting on them strangely and in a soulful way.

As the scotch continued to wear on, though, I became more depressed. Like I remembered that being excited about something sad and ambiguous didn't make sense. That Ethan and my ambitions were a poor tonic. And then I only wanted to go to bed, telling Ethan that I would. Like a good friend he saw the emotion written on my face, and with an understanding empathy said little, just sitting with me until I did. He sat with me as my face grew morose and the mixture of joy and melancholy blended together so that I could not tell the difference. I'm still not certain they aren't connected somehow.

THIRTY-TWO

WITH THOMAS AND ELIE GONE FOR THE WEEKEND, probably disrobed already in their room at the Pelican, Glower is down for another procedure. Apparently, the acid burned holes not only in his eyes but around them, and the tissue became infected. He's having a "debridement" as they call it in the fancy medical parlance of many syllables. Basically removing skin.

In all honesty and in spite of everything I'm doing well. At least in the sense that I know some outcome is going to be reached soon. In two days to be exact. I've spent the last few hours just kind of imagining what it will be like to have all my senses back. Being blind was fun for a while but I'm tired of it. Now, the other thing is I don't know if I'll regain the use of my body just because my mind is turned back on. Like all the muscle memory. To walk. To feed myself. To reel a trophy salmon, as the one that brought us here. I bet it'll be weird if it happens.

Two sets of footsteps enter. It's still the red-black that tells me it's morning.

"Are Marco's lawyers ready?"

"Yes, ma'am."

Regina has arrived with Ozzie, the latter tool having flown in from New York.

"And he's here in person?" Regina says.

"Yes, we took the same flight. He wanted to be on national television on Monday." Ozzie delivers this information as though he's reading the news. "He thinks being present for a medical miracle of sorts might boost his poll numbers," he goes on. "Genevieve is the better soldier in all this."

"Ed hasn't talked to him yet, has he?"

"No."

"I wonder what Genevieve said to him."

"I don't know."

"Well, Ed left quickly and meant business. It was ignorant to let Glower live." Regina pauses, glancing towards the hallway, "Wait, no, that wasn't him coming back. It was ignorant because look how much care he's inspiring here. What that could mean on Monday if he exposes us, to the world. Who knows who he's exposed us to already? I think Ed might kill him. He's a nurse and knows how. Just for his inheritance. But also to put him out of his misery. I think he also wants to uncover just how many lawyers Coraline has."

"I'll find him soon enough," Ozzie says.

"We'll sick the lawyers on them tomorrow. For now, stay with us. We've got a guest room."

"I can't," Ozzie says defiantly. "Genevieve gave me a message to give to Ed."

"And what's that?"

"I'd rather—"

"—I know Genevieve doesn't love the Governor, her husband," she says with thick innuendo. "She was all over Ed just recently, just like always, after he pledged his allegiance to us, and I know you're her bosom friend."

"Who, me?" Ozzie appears taken aback.

"I understand all of this. Look, my husband is dead, but we can't tell anyone how he broke his arm. Ed and I have talked and it's more convenient for Ed to be with me than with Genevieve. Like, she's still married, how ridiculous? Tell Ed *that* if you see him. And tell my sister to get her head straight. We'll see Glower when he's back, and you know what to do when you see him."

"You'll know who I'm with soon enough," Ozzie says, and departs. Several moments later Regina is gone, too.

"When are we going to be in my room?" Glower's voice arrives later that morning.

"We're here now," Ted's voice surprises me. Glower doesn't seem to know it's him, though, I suppose—imagining that he's homeless. I see Ted who says "Poor Tom" in my mind at once, flowing smoke in form and electric blue apertures of his soul.

"I thought we were still on the second floor. You're a good transporter," Glower says.

"No, we're here," Ted encourages. "Here, I'll open a window so you can hear the sea."

For a moment the shear brilliance of the Pacific Ocean, a thousand diamonds, as I've seen it so many times before, flashes before my eyes.

"I can't really hear it," Glower says.

"Your other senses must be growing imperfect due to your blindness," Ted speculates.

To be honest, I've wondered about that. The problem for me seems to be that all my senses save my hearing are impaired. Save my imagination, too, if you can call that a sense. I do. I can't tell if all my senses have been destroyed by my coma or if they've all been heightened. Some things seem more real than real, those visions of San Francisco, the three-dimensional figure of Lia I can see in my mind's eye, her beautiful button nose and almond eyes and curled hair. It makes me wonder about beauty itself, and how just having perfectly symmetric features by far doesn't capture what beauty is.

I can see her under a beam of light, angelic, her smooth skin when we were young, and how she's grown even more beautiful with age. All the imperfections the sign that she struggled, telling a story. Of never giving up. There's something more to beauty than just the way things look, too. Beauty is an action. A warmth. Something solid. And I'm wondering when I'll get my actions back. I'll change my actions if I get them back.

"Probably," Glower says. "Your voice sounds different from when we were downstairs."

Glower is absolutely right about that, too. I have a bit of a confession to make, that when I'm hearing my daughters and curious on-lookers, sometimes their voices are a little obscured. Or even like echoes.

"I'm the same," Ted says, perpetuating his ruse. I wonder if Glower can see the ghost who says "Poor Tom" as I can.

"You seem better spoken to me," Glower says.

"Perhaps. All I can tell you is that any day you see the ocean isn't a bad day," Ted says. "I can see sailboats like specks, like you know they're moving, except it's so slow you can't tell and they look stationary. Just past Ocean Beach. I see Cliff House as a doll house, and the people in Golden Gate Park look like ants. Somebody's down there picking flowers. It feels as though I might fall down there with them from up here."

Here, I'll put on a crown of flowers to go with my breathing tube, blood pressure cuff, and haggard lineaments. Just as we did in the '60s.

"Please, leave me alone here. I can see what you've described," Glower says. "Oh God," Glower continues after Ted in verbal cognito has left. "I'm sick of living in this world! I renounce all afflictions. If I could bear it I'd just let nature take me. Now, take me down to the ocean. If Ted's alive and no longer homeless, then God bless him!"

To make a confession, as I'm listening to this unfold my memories of my crown of flowers is dominating. As if it's happening now. Come with me. I'm wearing a crown of flowers. And a tie-dyed t-shirt, blue and red and purple and green, and we're smoking pot and Jimi Hendrix is playing Voodoo Chile on Hippie Hill and in Maui, lysergic acid diethylamide, lysergic acid die born by the tide, and I don't give a damn about anything. For I'm damned.

Don't I deserve this? Don't I deserve to return to a time and place where this nonsense doesn't make any sense and therefore it makes sense because it doesn't? Ah yes, I feel it all so clearly and coolly in my skin now. Like my entire body is being quickened by my crown of flowers. ZzzxZzzzxzip, zip! Hooray! Ha ha. Ha. Ha.

I'd never counterfeit money. I'm the CEO of everything.

Life breaks hearts better than any art can. Poor Tom, Thomas, Thomas Mariner, you are my recruit! Get your financing! Aim! Fire! Ha ha! I'm calling the lawyers. Genevieve and Regina falsely told me how great I was. Thinking it was how great a fortune they'd reap. And then when they stuck the tube down my throat, they wanted to pull it! Ha ha! When I had my seizure, I found out who they really were. ZzzzzxZxxxzzzz. They were lying when they told me how great I was. I had a seizure! Ha. Ha.

Yes, Glower. I'm a billionaire. A billion-aire. No heir. No air. No hair. No care. Billiion-aire. When I started making money, I became the most important person in the world. Not excrement, not a turd. Not disturbed. Nothing like what my father had carved out for me.

No. See? Glower! Hey! Glower! Did you cheat on your wife? Is that why you have two sons with the same name? Did you start over with a new family? Name both your sons the same? After you? Then they came and worked around you, because they thought you were something? Ha! I'll commute your sentence. To die for them. Your bastard son was more kind to you than my daughters are to me.

Go get busy again Glower, there's a hot young nurse waiting for you—I need workers in my company. See that nurse that comes in here in Parnassus? She acts like she's afraid of the word "sex," but she's hornier than a pack of polecats. She's a sex machine from the waist down, but discreet above her shoulders. You know what parts of her belong to God and which to the Devil!

Pharmacist! Where's my love perfume?! I've got one point six billion reasons for you.

Glower's got my hand. Somehow he's out of bed and over here. "Do you remember me?" He says, speaking directly to me. He alone knows I'm here. The first pilgrim. I try to link up in the other realm, but it's a lie. No. It's salvation. No. Damnation. "They've ruined you. Worn away to nothing."

No, Edward. I don't remember you. I do. Here, read this. Ha! You can't read! Thanks to Regina! Ha! Thanks to me. Thanks to thanks to thanks to thanks. Read it! Ha! You want me to pay you?! You won't read until your wallet is fat again?! I know you have less than you let on. Probably next to nothing. You bastards spend too much. Rich men like me don't admire your paltry pittance.

"I know you're in there, Steven," Glower says, his hand a calming presence. "I know you're afraid. I would be, too."

What, you're insane?! You can see how this wild world operates with no eyes! Look with your ears! I've been judging with my ears this whole time. Do you think the justice will be impartial to my daughters when he finds out you were maimed by them? That I was listening the whole time? That I was there? Have you ever seen dogs bark at Poor Tom? Poor Thomas, getting his right now at the Pelican. Getting his soul sucked dry by that lost one?

And you'll see him run. Run to the hills. Run run run run run run run to Chicago. To Washington. To New York. To Jim and Nick and

Anna. He'll run. After he's sucked dry. If he were mine I'd name him Danny all over again though he'd be different. Danny. Danny? Where are you? Did you hear me? Danny?! You won't join me in the other realm. Poor Tom, stop. Stop with that harlot. That strumpet. Don't punish her. It makes you a criminal just like them. Punishing each other. You are a poor man and your sins will always be more visible than theirs. Run, Poor Tom! Run, Ted! Run, run, RUN, HA! They'll cover up their crimes with gold, but you'll need tennis shoes. And don't let your clothes become rags. They'll find you. Just like they found me. AND THEY DIDN'T FIND MY FATHER!

Everyone commits crimes. Glower, get two glass eyes and pretend to see things like Dumb Dom, like Marco Brouwer, that corrupt politician.

Suddenly the ghost who says "Poor Tom" appears in front of me, an insane apparition. "You're wise," he says, with those blue beams into my soul. "Reason in madness!"

How do you know what you know? Why is there something and not nothing?

I'm a newborn. I'm a newborn. I'm a little baby. I have to start all over, just like I'm a little baby. Do you want my eyes so you can cry, Glower? We come into this world crying, the first whiff we get. Cry! Let me sermonize. We come into this world and cry to be amongst fools, Dumb Dom, Dumb Dom, do you hear me?! I'll kill kill kill kill kill!!!

THIRTY-THREE

"I BELIEVE HE HAD A MILD SEIZURE," GLOWER SAYS TO the brainwave technologist. "I could tell holding his hand."

I'm tired, but not as after the seizure I suffered at St. Mary's. What did I just say? Can anyone listening tell me what I just said? I only vaguely remember. A bad trip.

"We'll only connect him over the weekend."

Great, the goop and the electrodes are back. And at the behest of a blind man.

"It will help us know what to expect on Monday," Glower concludes.

I do believe I'll wake up. But if I do, it will be from the cell I've inhabited. Are our cranial vaults not cells? Our senses our only way out. And what are my senses? What of my processing? My language? I remain afraid of what I just said.

Was I offering to sling money? I sometimes offer to sling money when I'm afraid. I believe Glower is perceptive. Even without eyes.

I remember when I was first imagining the money I would make. And the life I would live afterwards. I had an edge. Every need would be met. People everywhere. All day. Every day. That I paid. For Lia and my future home in Sea Cliff. The same place we'd raise our kids. Just down the street, where Danny first laid eyes on Elie. And where Thomas is living with her.

And it happened. Lawyers everywhere, protecting our fortune, as they are now. Finance men, tending to and expanding the fortune through investment. Ventures. NDAs. People there to protect us as they took from us. The ecosystem I'd built.

But also: what power. What power I felt I would come into. My son-in-law the governor of New York. The other a California Reagan. Lia and I sat in box seats at the theatre across the street from City Hall every season. That ancestral play of my obsession. Over and over again. The pinnacles of culture.

What will become of my becoming? Was it tremendous and good of me, or a blind descent with disastrous consequences?

We—I—continue descending. Whereas in the past my journey began with Kim to the center of my consciousness, I feel stuck now. Or perhaps not stuck, but merely as though a dam is ready to break. The pressure is bearable, but the door begins to splinter. I tried to let it in, but the numbing let it build up. Until there was a mad mob outside, pitchforks in hand, ready to break down my door, put me in the stocks, feather me. If I'd only kept descending. They wouldn't be here. I'd be out of their reach. Though even despite this, I'll die with courage.

For now, I'm going. My head is light. My dreams have deposited me here. Borne by the tide. I feel true sleep will arrive soon.

THIRTY-FOUR

SOMEHOW I FELT BETTER FOR FEELING WORSE. THAT I would perhaps never know what truly happened or the motivations for it tore down my guard like nothing ever had. I was left to accept I might always be left me with so many questions. Like why had my father acted the way he had, rather than just tell me the truth? Perhaps he'd never journeyed to the center of his consciousness about it. He didn't know what really happened either, as Harry said, and that's why he couldn't talk about it. Whether he was conscious of it or not didn't matter.

"You ready?" Were Ethan's first words the next morning as we ate breakfast of scrambled eggs and reindeer sausage.

"Yeah," I said, petting Nali. "Ready for anything."

"Good," he said. "Because weather says a storm is coming. We've got about fifty miles to survey before the end of next week. Garland Pass. Going to be an early winter this year." It was late September. "If we make it in time, we'll miss the weather. No promises. We'll need to take gear," he said. I could tell by the fact that he wasn't as maniacal describing potentially dangerous events that it concerned him.

"And what if we don't make it in time?"

"Well, the bank is threatening to withdraw their funding," he said.

"What?" I was shocked.

"You could say I stretched the timeline a little. They thought we'd be a little closer to Anchorage by now. That we'd already be laying pipe. They've got a lot of people begging for money, and we're slipping on their list," he said, with a hint of urgency glossed over with confidence.

Great, I thought, recoiling. *After coming all this way, even my fortune was in question. On account of my unreliable friend who'd lied to the banks, and an early snowstorm. Two things I couldn't have predicted.*

We urgently packed most of the day.

"We'd better go," I said. It was reaching late afternoon.

"We'll leave first thing," Ethan's confidence was nearing nonchalance. He had that kind of confidence where you believed him just because he was so assured.

"Whatever you say," I sounded annoyed. Though inside giving myself to whatever outcome was reached.

The next morning we packed up his Jeep with the tents we'd need, as well as a few firearms for protection and possibly if we ran out of food, Ethan joked. We were going to drive about an hour east and then south of Fairbanks, through a stretch of country known as Garland Pass, which featured a valley through which the pipeline would need to travel somehow.

"I figure we might need to drill some tunnels," Ethan said as we entered the dirt road portion of our drive, Nali in the back seat and dust rising behind us like smoke. "For it to make sense. They had to do the same thing with the railroad."

"Is Fluor prepared for that kind of engineering project?" I asked.

"Well, we'd better be," he said, lighting a cigarette.

I hated smoking though couldn't resist. "Mind if I bum one of those?"

"Sure," he opened the aluminum container.

"Are we meeting anyone there?"

"A guy from corporate is coming behind us. I kind of need him to vouch that we're going to make it through the pass. The banks want to know, as well, and they'll believe him."

"You're using someone from corporate?" I asked.

"Listen, man," Ethan said, again soulfully, almost as if his soul was asserting dominance over my doubts, "—I am corporate. We're working as a team. We're going to be fine."

We arrived at our destination a little after mid-day, as the road became worse, like it typically did the farther you went into the bush. Potholes the size of basketballs and just about as deep, we had to slink across the road in places to find just level terrain. The sky was clearing up so the clouds looked like chicken scratch. Just high, harmless wisps.

"So far so good," Ethan said, referring to the terrain and not necessarily anything to do with our situation. "Nothing we can't get over. It's the valley they're worried about."

Garland Pass is legendary to the people of Fairbanks, both as a playground during the summers but also as a marking post for those traveling north. Some of the largest inland grizzlies could be found there due to the abundant food supplies in the non-winter months, and one would be liable to see dall sheep, moose, lynx, wolves, beavers, and any number of other wild creatures. It was said during the prospecting days that once you'd reached it you were more than half way there. And if one were able to cross it, they would be at the starting point. The starting point was for the Brooks Range of mountains, situated dead in the center of the state. Garland Pass had taken on a mythical quality for me, as I'd never been but heard a lot about it.

"How exactly are we supposed to tell them it's safe or not?" I asked, as we descended into the valley, crisscrossing down a steep slope.

"That's right," Ethan said. "You've only done flat-land surveying up until this point. Bottom line is we had instruments that tell us certain angles. It's our job to prove there's at least one path the pipeline can take. Even if it means . . . " and he continued to describe the process by which the tunnels might be created.

I could tell Ethan was nervous. I didn't let it bother me. Again, I felt I had nothing worse to fear, having just reached the point I had with the situation with my father. In fact, as we continued our about-face descent, I even began to feel a little joy, even pleasure. Not only for the excitement of what it all could mean, but some kind of peace entered my chest and spread throughout my body, a warm kind of buzzing, as I reached back and petted Nali. Who licked my forearm as I did.

"Why don't we stop here," he said, as we came to a kind of open plane in the valley. The crown of the mountains surrounded us and I began to imagine how people had crossed with just horses once upon a time. How much had changed.

The valley itself hadn't. A slight wind had picked up and there was a soft laughter that you could hear in it, as it whisked through the low-growing trees. Not a mirthful laughter either. Something that every Alaskan knew at one point or another, though. A kind of baiting to push the limits of survival. Like Ethan and I were doing now.

A moose and calf entered the forest in the distance. "Let's get to work," Ethan said, unloading the surveying instruments, including a tripod and a camera. "We're burning daylight."

We finished unpacking the remainder of our gear which included a plastic tub full of camp food, snowshoes if need be, a small gas range, the guns, and our tent. The latter which we decided to pitch that evening. We got to work setting up the instruments and Ethan did most of the work.

"I always thought the pipe should come through the northern-most foothill's midpoint," Ethan said. "It'll allow a lesser gradient descent for the pipeline to come through the valley. That's the easy part."

"What's it called, again?" I remembered the peak's had names.

"Ipalook," Ethan lent.

"The southern you thinking the same?" I asked. I remembered it was named "Tikaani", the Athabaskan word for "wolf."

"Probably similarly," he said. "Though if this thing—" he pointed the surveying instruments in that direction and adjusted the camera, "—if this thing is correct the slope is slightly steeper. The tunnel might need to begin closer to the base and angle up more gradually."

The wind was really starting to pick up, blowing the tent in its container so that the outer plastic coating rippled.

"The question is where to lead the pipe in and where out," he said over the wind. "That's what we need to figure."

You could see down the valley as the mountains were corrugated before sloping around to the east, meaning there were multiple paths. The valley itself was probably seven miles across, which meant we would need to take detailed pictures and measurements of everything.

"So far so good," Ethan said again, as we roasted chicken breasts after making camp, crackling on the gas grill inside our tent, the multiple stakes we'd planted keeping it and the tents from blowing away in the growing wind. Which groaned and whistled. "But you know this means something's on its way." His face appeared lit from the gas grill alone, so that his eye sockets seemed like craters with two shining stars. Nali had her fill and was laying contentedly on her side.

"We need to haul you know what tomorrow, with any luck we'll finish day after tomorrow and beat the worst of it," he concluded.

"What's the back-up plan?" I said. "In case we don't finish."

He looked at me as if that were a ridiculous question.

I awoke in the middle of the night, surprised to hear the wind had died down. My recollection was this was either a good or bad thing, considering the wind had come from the southwest, and meant that whatever pattern was coming was either almost here, or simply perhaps stalled.

I lay there for probably thirty minutes, unable to sleep. I could hear Ethan and Nali in deep repose. I imagined some of my awakening was subliminal. Some kind of delayed adrenaline. I rolled over in my down sleeping bag, unable to fall back asleep. I imagined it must have been three in the morning. Rather than just lay there, I decided to get up and go outside. Maybe steal a cigarette from Ethan, have a granola bar.

Instead, emerging from the tent I bore witness to the most awe-inspiring tableau in the sky you could possibly imagine. I'd forgotten it was the season when you could start seeing the aurora borealis, or "northern lights" as some people call them. I hadn't seen them since I was fourteen years old or so. And never like this.

It seemed whatever wind had blown away the cloud cover of that day, and the moon was brilliant white, peaking just above the Ipalook slope to the north, illuminating the perfectly still terrain, short and taller pines a few hundred yards to the north and south. But the sky. The sky!

Phosphorescent green, blue, and purple, electric and metallic, the flow of the atmosphere dancing against darkness. As if to music. A little kid begging for you to play with it. My eyes were fixed, unable to avert my gaze from the most spectacular display I'd ever witnessed. For a brief minute, I forgot everything. Suffused. Nothing mattered. Only what was in front of me, above me. Like the first time I kissed Lia, I wanted to escape to spaces where the depth of what I felt—what I felt at what I saw—could be commensurate. As the colors flowed together creating a photic estuary, their movement caused the white illumination of the moon to change color as well, so that I could see these greens, azures, purples color my cheeks. On my arms. Shifting across the permafrost.

I couldn't bring myself to light a cigarette and spoil it, so I just sat down on a fallen tree trunk about fifteen feet from our tent. Simply awed. For the better part of a half hour. My neck was the only thing that stopped me, as it grew tired. And then my whole body, like whatever adrenaline I'd felt, all that I'd stored from what I'd been through in pursuit of the truth about my past, all of it washed away. And I felt as though it was time to go back to sleep. I took a granola bar out of the plastic tub, which we kept suspended on a tree branch with a pulley system to avoid any animals getting into it.

As I finished pulling the rope to re-suspend the plastic tub, I saw round tracks greater than the size of a human hand with five toes and the prints of claws pressed into the mud.

THIRTY-FIVE

"I DON'T KNOW WHAT I COULD EVER DO TO MATCH what you've done for my father over the past few weeks," Coraline says to Ken. They've come to my bedside at early red-black o'clock. Glower is away at yet another procedure. This time to ensure the sockets of his eyes heal properly.

"To have it acknowledged is enough," Ken says.

"I hope you can wear your long white coat again soon," Coraline encourages, apparently having heard of Ken's former banishment from the residency program.

"Not until after Monday," he says. "If I'm known as a resident from St. Mary's and UCSF, my intentions will be thwarted. Please don't talk to me in front of the cameras on Monday until I tell you."

"Whatever you need," Coraline agrees. "How is my father?"

"He's still sleeping," Ken says.

"Oh God," Coraline laments, unable to suppress her emotion at this persistent truth. "Please cure his illness. At how his children have driven him crazy to an infantile state."

"We could see if he'll wake up now," Ken says, sensing action may assuage her bereavement. "It might actually be a good thing to keep him somewhat stimulated before Monday. If he wakes up, great. If not, he'll be primed. As of today, he's been comatose a long time."

"Do what you believe is best," Coraline agrees to have Ken torture me again. "I only wish that the nation could see him on Monday in his proper CEO's clothes."

"We had to put him in the gown," Ken speaks with an apologetic tone. "But here, come closer," Ken encourages her.

She takes a few, slow steps. Silence. Then I feel Coraline lean over and kiss me on my forehead.

"Oh, Daddy," she says, "—Daddy. I hope the medicine works, whatever they're going to do to you on Monday. What violence they did by not respecting you. They would've treated a stranger better." She kisses me again. Then suddenly she reaches her hand onto Ken's arm, "I think he's waking…!! Talk to him…!!"

"He recognizes your voice," Ken says, as I stir, my eyes open, seeing again the dark shapes. "It makes more sense for you to…"

"Daddy, how are you? Dad?!"

Coraline, I feel wronged by your trying to take me from the grave. You're an angel, while these tears on the bitten ventilator tube burn my face in hell, I say to myself.

"Do you know it's me?!" Her voice rises as the shapes again fade to red-black.

I see your spirit, Coraline you are a spirit, I continue.

"He's gone again," Coraline says to Ken.

Oh God, where have I been? Where am I? Is it daylight or night? I have journeyed still closer to the center of my consciousness, and I am beginning to see the rift open up, like the San Andreas fault. I am ready to enter. To burn to see what is at the center. Oh, I have come close. So close.

"Give a thumbs up, Steve," Ken says again, for old times.

I'm afraid I'm losing my sanity again. Like my ears aren't connected to my eyes, that my words aren't connected to my tongue. That I should recognize Ken's spirit, and Coraline's—for some reason I can only sense Ken's. Am I in France?

"What will we do when . . . if he wakes up?" Coraline asks.

"We have no reason to believe he'll be altered. Disoriented, yes, so it will probably be best not to ask him too many questions. He may have regressed. Some people return to themselves slowly. It depends. Give it time."

"Will he be able to walk?" Coraline continues.

"All in time. There's a chance. We don't know for sure how much damage will be evident. The device is only proven to help him regain consciousness."

"Is it true that Dominic, my brother-in-law, is dead?

"That's what I've heard."

"With charges filed our lawyers will meet in arbitration soon," Coraline insinuates.

"I've heard Ed, Glower's illegitimate son, is with your sisters' attorneys," Ken says.

"Everything depends on Monday," Coraline says, her voice trembling. "If he's able to settle this for us."

"Is there anything else I can help you with?" Ken says. "I need to be going, I have to give a didactic session at lunch."

"I should be, as well," Coraline says. "Thank you again. We'll see you soon."

It is now Saturday afternoon, I believe. A mere thirty-six hours until I awake from my long slumber. In some regards I will be emerging a different man. What lessons I have learned while sleeping. Too many to recount. The most important ones centered in what is genuine and what is artificial. I know I will change.

I again sense Danny is on his way, probably boarding in Kabul. Is he on a cargo plane, or something more comfortable? I'm sure he doesn't care. I sense that he is worried about me and wants to take me somewhere. Maybe he wants to take me fishing. Maybe he wants to take me with him when he runs his first political campaign. As a veteran. Like me.

What will Lia look like when I wake up? I bet she looks every bit as magnetic and angelic as she has our entire lives together. She is the strongest, smartest, most radiant, sensitive, cunning, tender, loving human being to ever grace the planet. A beacon of light in a world of darkness, and I hope that her face is the first thing I see. If I am able to speak, I will say that I love her a thousand times before I say anything else. And with Danny there I imagine I'll be overwhelmed with pure joy.

I hear one set of footsteps enter. Unfamiliar footsteps. Furtive footsteps.

"Steve," Ferris says, addressing me not as 'Mr. Levinson' kind of disrespectfully. "Steve, you're going to make me a millionaire. Many times over." He approaches the bed, and I can feel the sliminess of his mirth, his pallid and drained face. "I've gotten to know Dr. Gideon quite well, quite well," he continues. "And when the country sees what he invented . . . bring a billionaire back to life; well, it's game over. I'm a CEO now, just like you—" his voice grows thicker and more sinister, "—just like you. And the market for 'the quickening device', as Gideon calls it, is large, all over the world. And when Danny gets here, he won't have any idea that I'm using all of you, including the good doctor, just to prove a point. Thomas has no idea what's coming for him either. I told Carmelia Danny is going to propose, to make you what you are: an outcast. And then, I know a guy in North Beach who told me he killed a man for fifty dollars. I asked him if he'd do it for free. And he said 'yes'—" he laughs, out loud. "—He said 'yes'. And soon. Very soon. Danny will have to get over it, too, and you'll understand, when Elie sees what I've done—brought you and countless others back to life—and when she finally sees this and the money I've made as a result, she'll reject Danny. For good.

And when she and I are taking our kids up to the mountain house in Tahoe, we'll send you a postcard. Thank you, Steve. For how beautiful all this will be. For me."

I really hate this kid.

THIRTY-SIX

AS THE WIND BEGAN TO CREEP UP AGAIN THE FOLLOWing morning, I decided not to tell Ethan about the footprints I'd seen the previous night. As I mentioned before, by this point I was kind of resigned to anything, and this was why I was also nonchalant about telling Ethan about the bear. Ethan fed Nali and I had a quick breakfast of a few granola bars.

"With any luck we'll get to the other end of the pass by three o'clock," Ethan said. "We're going to need to be perfect. The storm shouldn't arrive until this evening, if the predictions I heard are correct."

"What about the other Fluor people? Are they still meeting us?"

"If they get here. They were supposed to be here by now. I'm not sure what the hold-up is. Anyway, they don't know I plan to finish today. This'll surprise them," he said with that wild and soulful look enlivening his eyes.

We should take a brief moment to remember that this was 1973, and we had no way of communicating with the outside world. No GPS. No cellphones. We really were taking a chance on our wits. I just kind of took it for granted that they were sound.

Then something happened that we both weren't expecting. And that was that Nali started to run away, towards the Northern, Ipalook side of the valley. For no reason.

"Nali!" Ethan shouted, as she retreated farther and farther away, towards where we'd seen the moose and its calf. "Nali, come back!" starting to run after her. But she kept running. "God dammit!!" he shouted, exasperated after about fifty yards of chasing. She ran and ran and didn't look back.

"Nali!!" I called after him in futility.

"It's the damn wolf in her," he said. "I was afraid this would happen," with emotion thickening his voice.

"Should we drive after her?" I asked.

"No," he said, appearing deflated. "We can't get back in those trees. We don't have time, anyway."

"I'm sorry man," I said, trying to console.

"Let's keep going," Ethan looked more defeated than I'd ever seen him.

We did as he said, as we had to, parking in the next clearing.

"That's another part of the slope I think we could come down. The problem is where on the southern end," he said, as I set up the tripod, as he prepared the camera and its measuring instruments. "There's good, flat terrain through here." Which is why we'd stopped in this location.

Taking the measurements with the camera took the better part of half an hour, even with this frenetic pace. Ethan said little, and his thick breath began creating plumes of smoke as the temperature began to drop precipitously around eleven a.m. As we packed the tripod to move to our next position, another two miles down the canyon, it began to feel as though it was a minute away from snowing.

"We're making good time," Ethan said, as the inside of the windshield began to fog over so that we had to turn the defroster on, with jets of warm air coming from deep vents.

We entered a part of the road that wasn't really a road, if you could even call it that. This part of the pass was so unfrequented by humans that it was really more a bumpy, grassed-over trail which led into increasingly thickening woods. Around eleven o'clock the wind began rushing at us and swirling all around, so that you could hear it through that window.

"This is going to make our job more difficult," Ethan said again, dispassionately, probably sensing my withdrawal. Normally we'd be talking if not howling like the current wind, about old times. The thing with Nali had hurt us both, him more than me.

"Is there any way we can cut corners?" I asked. "Not because we want to, but because we have to?"

"Not really," he said. "I mean, we need to get pretty precise angles of the slope and all the terrain, which requires at least a dozen measurements in each direction. I guess I can try to go faster, but with the consequences being that oil spills out into the pass…"

"Well, can we take measurements at the same time?" I asked, thinking maybe if we doubled up, we'd have a better chance.

Ethan stopped to consider, and I could tell he'd done this type of thing—the dual measurements—before.

"Not really," he said again. "But I don't think we have a choice."

I exhaled, my breath a thick frost.

"At our next stop," he said, "take the back-up camera. You use the tripod because you've got less experience. I'll take surveys of Tikanni, you do Ipalook."

"Okay."

As we got out of the jeep after bumping our way into a wooded area, finally arriving at a small clearing, it felt like the wind was gusting a hundred miles an hour. I'd taken measurements like these north of Fairbanks, near the Yukon River, though never for a canyon the likes of Garland Pass. I began to lose faith in what we were doing as first snowflakes started to flurry all around us.

"Ethan," I said directly, as he finished his portion. It was now approaching two o'clock. "Do you think it's worth it?"

"If you want our financing, yes," he said. "The bank told me they're ready to pull out if we're not done by the end of the year. There's going to be no chance of coming back after this storm. So yes."

Again, while I may have wanted to, I couldn't argue. Something about there only being flurries seemed to belie what was coming, as well.

"All right," I said. "How many more stops? How the hell are we going to make it out today?"

"Two more," he said. And by my calculations, that meant at least an hour more driving and at least another hour of measurements, which meant we'd be turning around to leave probably by four o'clock. That would also mean driving back across the canyon, through the bad "roads". There was no way we'd be out before seven or eight o'clock, right in the middle of whatever was coming.

"Let's go," I said.

We all but tumbled forward, the forest growing thicker and then thinning again, before we came to the second to last clearing, the second to last viable route for the pipeline to traverse Garland Pass. Snow began falling thicker flurries, the kind of snow that starts to accumulate. Ethan got the tripod out again and handed it to me as we planned to reprise what we'd just done in the last clearing. Just a dozen or so measurements to take.

Something strange happened then, though. Even though the wind was gusting and taking flurries every direction with it—up, down, and swirling around us and making a considerable noise—as I set the tripod down, I heard what sounded like a crack in the woods about a hundred yards to the north, where I was facing the tripod. Initially I just kind of blew it off as the wind causing a branch to fall. But I was wrong.

I took the first measurement of the peak of an Ipalook slope ridge, where we might burrow the tunnel. But right after that I heard something that sounded like a sneeze except much deeper, through a gust of wind. Then another crack.

"Ethan," I said. "Ethan!" I shouted.

As he turned towards me his eyes grew wide at the sight of an inland grizzly bear, not more than fifty yards away from us. It took me back instantly to the day with the wolf-dog when we were children, though this was a less domesticated predator.

"Raise your arms!" Ethan shouted at me, giving the advice you give people who don't know that for grizzly bears you're first supposed to make yourself ominous. The bear was walking at us at a slow, steady pace, knowing it could outrun both of us if we chose to go.

I don't know how to describe what I felt in that moment other than sheer terror. And stupidity. Why hadn't I told Ethan what I saw the night before? It would have at least given him the chance to load the firearms, which he slowly walked towards the back of the jeep to find, as they were propped up against the locked trunk.

"Hey!" I shouted. "Hey!" raising my arms and waving them back and forth. Nothing. The bear just kept slowly sauntering towards us, nonchalant. I supposed he was a juvenile. Though, as he came in full view, I saw scars on his shoulders from encounters with other bears. I realized he was older. "Hey!" I doubled down. "We're going to shoot you!"

The bear only picked up his pace at my words, now thirty yards, then twenty away, before stopping to sniff something quickening the frigid air as the snow then grew thicker. "Ethan!" I shouted.

"The aught six is frozen," he said, terrified. "I can't get it open!"

He ran towards the front door and tried to open it, as well. "It's frozen shut, too," Ethan all but screamed. Then I really panicked.

"Let's play dead!" Ethan said calmly, as the bear resumed its slow saunter towards us. The idea is that if the bear thinks you're already dead—grizzly bears, anyway—that if they think you're already dead, they'll leave you alone. Black bears will eat you regardless, as they're not so well-fed. This one was probably just defending its territory, I reassured myself. It was incredibly fat from eating so much prior to hibernating and didn't want another meal.

I laid on the ground, with Ethan only a few feet from me, towards the trunk, where our frozen guns were. "Don't move," Ethan said under his breath.

I didn't, as the bear was now a mere forty feet away, walking slowly. I wanted to cry but knew I couldn't, because dead things can't cry. Each footstep I heard, as its padded foot thudded on the cold Earth. I was sure I was a few moments away from death.

I closed my eyes as the bear snorted several times, and for the first time I smelled the thick, pungent smell of a live grizzly. I'd never been nor ever wanted to be this close. I made a small slit with my right eye as its face was now a foot from mine, and I held my breath as its own, warm maw opened and it moaned a low grumble of saliva on my forehead. A roar to let me know who ruled this place. I told myself I was ready.

But then its face backed away. Sensing my demise Ethan made a whooping sound, startling the bear momentarily. It backed away slowly, going over nearer the jeep, standing up on its hind quarters to inspect what was inside. For the time being our simple ploy seemed to work. The bear sniffed and snorted near Ethan, though from what I could tell it wasn't interested in him either.

It then began rocking the jeep back and forth, smelling the open plastic food container, the same one it had probably tried to infiltrate the night before. As it did Ethan looked over at me and I at him, both laid out on the frozen tundra, lightly dusted with snow. The bear continued rocking the jeep, now with such force that it rolled over on its side, glass breaking and crashing.

The bear I could then see was probably twelve feet tall, and probably weighted fourteen hundred pounds. It rocked the jeep one more time until all the side windows were broken. It then dug its face into the car, grabbing the food container with its teeth, our lunch and dinner strewn across the forest floor. It began eating the leftover chicken, tearing at the bread and granola bars, taking bites of apples and smoked salmon, devouring Nali's dried beef.

This went on for what seemed like an eternity. But was probably less than ten minutes. Ethan and I laid still and it seemed the bear wasn't interested in us anymore. Maybe we didn't smell right. When it was satisfied that it had everything the car had to offer, it began a slow departure. Just as nonchalant as when it had approached.

When it was forty feet from us, though, we made a mistake. I looked over at Ethan and he mouthed the words "Let's run" to me. I nodded. And before an instant we did.

But it was a mistake for two reasons. Number one, bears, like that wolf dog, also have a "chase instinct", meaning that anything smaller than it that's running seems automatic prey. And so we were. The second mistake was not waiting until it was gone gone, thinking we could outrun a bear, even of its size. The damned things can run up to twenty miles per hour. Though somehow, and I'm not sure if it was just that all the blood was drained from our brains, or we were just so traumatized, but we started running.

"Go-go-go-go-go-go-go-go-go," Ethan shouted as we ran together through thickening snowfall.

The bear took note. We got a decent head start on it. Except even after only thirty or forty yards at the speed we could run as twenty somethings, I started wondering where the hell were we running. "Where are we going?!" I yelled.

"Just go!" Ethan shouted.

"Let's climb a tree!" I shouted back, just behind him. The bear was pursuing us in a slow gallop now and I could hear the cracking of branches as we made our way through the flurries and the forest. I figured we had time to climb something, though the trees were relatively low.

"Here!" Ethan shouted after another twenty or thirty yards, finding a spruce tree.

The branches were low enough that we could both get our arms on the lowest hanging ones, and even though I was getting scratched and cut on my hands, I pulled myself up, as Ethan made his way. We'd need to get at least twelve feet up to avoid the bear, as grizzlies aren't known for climbing.

Its slow gallop intensified, faster, as I got my foothold on the lowest branch, probably five feet in the air. The bear arrived and swiped at Ethan, clawing his leg as he made his way out of its reach. I remained unscathed but for the spruce needles stinging my face, as we both made it about half way up the tree.

The bear stood on all fours at the base and again made a moaning sound. And something of several woofs, again as if stating who was in charge of Garland Pass. I don't know if it really wanted to eat us or if it simply wanted to kill us. It hung around for another fifteen minutes.

"Come and get us, you bastard!" Ethan taunted. Due to the adrenaline, he didn't realize his leg was dripping blood on the forest floor.

"We're waiting!" I echoed.

Eventually though the bear's kill instinct dissipated. It woofed and moaned again as it made its final retreat, having treed its rivals. I had never felt so helpless in all my life. Not even in Vietnam.

"We'll have to stay here a while," Ethan said, inspecting his leg. He had three claw marks that had gone through his blue jeans, which were tattered to his mid-calf. "There won't be a next time if he sees us."

I thought to myself that with the snow intensifying there might not be a next time for anything, anyway.

"You're a genius for grabbing the aught six," Ethan said, noting what I'd done as we'd taken off.

"I'm not sure doing something smart in the middle of something stupid makes a person smart," I said.

The snow was now really coming down, so that you couldn't see more than twenty or thirty yards away. The only thing we had going for us was that we both had down winter jackets on, and aside Ethan's torn jeans we were both wearing gloves, long underwear and wool socks with thickly insulated boots.

"What the hell are we going to do?" I said out loud after half an hour of the thicker snowfall.

"Let's not talk about that right now," Ethan said, with his soulful tone returning.

"We're going to die," I finally let the emotion get to me. It was getting on in the evening and we were stuck in the tree.

"No, we're not," Ethan said. "I'm not."

And I'm not sure where his confidence came from. For some reason while I thought I was being more realistic, it occurred to me that you truly don't have a chance unless you think you do. As I'm thinking right now, before Monday.

The snow accumulated for the next several hours on every branch and spare patch of clearing. I didn't have a ruler but had measuring on the mind and so imagined that we'd received at least a foot by the middle of the night, as the cold began to get to me.

"Well, we got ourselves in another situation," Ethan said as twilight set in.

"You could call it that," I said.

"If only we'd known to climb a tree when we were kids, running from that she-wolf."

We both laughed a little.

"We had some pretty wild times when we were kids," I said. "Doesn't seem like that long ago."

"It sure doesn't," Ethan said, meaning it.

"What's your old man up to now, besides Fluor?" I asked.

"Mainly flying his plane. Occasionally taking my Mom to Hawaii," Ethan said, soulful again.

"Ah," I returned.

"What about your folks. Well, I shouldn't ask." He paused for a moment, seeing what I'd say. When I didn't say anything, he said, "Do you think he really doesn't know?"

"Yes," I said.

"Well, you'll have to take it up with him someday." Ethan had a way of putting things to bed that were difficult, a way that gave you confidence you could handle them. About this it was no different.

"What do you think you'll do with the money we make, if we make it out of here alive?" I asked him.

"I'm not sure," he said, as if he hadn't thought about it. That seemed the problem with so many of my efforts, I thought. Things I did because I could, not because I knew why. "I think I'll probably move south. Or at least get a place. You enjoying San Francisco?"

"Very much," I said.

"What are you going to do?"

I stopped to think. What had gone on recently had kind of scrambled my priorities, as important hidden things will do. It wasn't long before I knew what I wanted to say.

"There's a girl from my hometown named Lia," I said. "That's what I'm going to do."

"Oh, man," Ethan said, laughing. "You're smitten."

"Like a wise man once told me: don't settle down until you find someone who makes you want to settle down. And she does," I said.

"Why?" He asked.

"I'll tell you when it's official," I said, instead of saying 'if we survive' again. I was beginning to feel optimistic. I stopped for a second to think. "And after talking with Harry Frank, that guy in Fairbanks, I'll probably start a fishing business in the Queen Charlotte Islands—or Haida Gwai, as they called it first—someday. That's the tribe he's a member of."

"The Charlottes are awesome," Ethan said. "I'll go on one of your trips."

By this point the snow had stopped falling and the clouds were also beginning to pass over us. The sky was dark and holding in the night. The stars were out, but there were no northern lights. A bright, waxing gibbous moon shone across Garland Pass, reflecting soft white light that caused the snow to glow and sparkle, soft and luminescent, dimly glowing on every living creature. Dark silence. There was a ravine about twenty yards to the north and the shape of the snow made it look like a frozen river of glowing, powdered sand.

"We might as well try to get some sleep," Ethan said. "There's no chance we make it out tonight."

"I agree," I said. I felt comfortable sitting on my limb except that the exposed parts of my face had grown a little numb. The adrenaline had worn off and I was suddenly exhausted. "I could sleep right here."

"We'll get out in the morning," he said, yawning. And again I couldn't help but believe him.

"Good night, Ethan," I said after a few minutes, leaning my head on my arms which were perched on a branch in front of me.

"'Night, Steve," Ethan returned, doing the same.

THIRTY-SEVEN

I AWOKE TO THE CRASHING OF SNOW ON MY HEAD, SO that it both startled me and shocked me awake. When that much snow accumulates in that short a time, it's inevitable that the trees are going to start shedding it by the slightest wind. It was morning and the wind had picked up again. The clouds had returned in short order and it felt as it had at noon the day before. The crashing snow woke Ethan, as well.

"Shit," he said.

"Better than morning coffee," I joked.

"All right," Ethan continued. "It's time we get out of here."

How that was going to happen I wasn't sure. Only that Ethan had a plan. We climbed down from the fifteen or so feet we were up in the tree, and I was actually feeling somewhat refreshed. Something about my warm clothes and the sleeping in the cold elements. My body was tired, however, fatigued from the past forty-eight hours.

"We're going to have to walk," he said, kind of insinuating that the jeep had been totaled.

We crunched our way through a foot of snow, so that it felt as though the five or so miles we needed to walk was like twenty. Compounded by intense hunger and the returning elements, I began to wonder if we'd both make it.

"How's your leg?" I asked Ethan.

"It's too numb to really feel the pain right now," was all he said.

We crunched a short way back to the road and smaller, maybe fifty-yard clearing.

"Shit," Ethan said. "I'm already turned around." The northern and southern slopes were easy enough, though he meant finding the road.

"I think we went too far south," I said. "I think we need to go back north, maybe twenty, thirty yards."

"Okay," he said, assenting.

As we retraced our steps, I leading Ethan, however, I heard a moan come from behind us. That again wasn't human. We both turned and I reflexively began preparing the aught six, which I'd pried open overnight. It appeared the bear had waited us out. It *did* want two more tastes of meat. In short order it revealed itself, not fifty yards to the south.

"Oh God," Ethan said.

In that moment I loaded the chamber of the aught six with a shell, then another. The bear began its nonchalant saunter towards us. I froze, with the aught six weighing on my hands, looking at Ethan between me and the approaching predator.

Here I was. I had my chance. The bear had taken our food but the measurements were going to be sufficient. All I had to do was take the shot. It was like everything was moving in slow motion. I looked at Ethan. The bear. I didn't know what to do. Ethan was speaking. I couldn't hear him. I couldn't run. I couldn't think. There I was. Ready with my shot. All I had to do was take it.

THIRTY-EIGHT

IT WAS SUNDAY AND THE STEPS I HEARD ENTER THAT morning, I think my mind was primed for them to sound like rubber boots. I guess because that's what I expected Danny to arrive in. But they weren't. It sounded like a pair of heels and shoes similar to Glower's former clopping.

"We just need to make a few final preparations before tomorrow," Dr. Eugene says.

"Like what?" Lia asks.

"Well, the pulmonologists have him on a breathing trial," she continues. And for the first time I realize that the ventilator isn't controlling my breath. It feels fine. "It's actually a prerequisite to anything we'll do. We've done it before. The breathing tube has to come out before we try the device."

"Okay," Lia says agreeably.

"Is your son going to be here?" Eugene asks.

"As far as I know," Lia says. "He's military, and supposedly on a plane to see us right now. I haven't spoken to him for a week, but he told me he'd be here."

"Because at this point we can't wait," Eugene says, measured and calm.

"I understand," Lia says.

"And I've heard there will be quite a few others," Eugene says. "We'll need their names prior."

"Thomas Mariner, Eleanor Monroe, Ferris Bundy and his father—"

"—You don't have to tell me everyone today. We'll write them down. With the media here we just want to make sure no one unauthorized makes it in."

"Understood," Lia says.

"Lia, you do understand there's a good chance he'll wake up," Eugene encourages.

"I understand."

"Because we haven't talked about all the possibilities. Have you spoken with palliative care?"

"We don't have to," she says. "And yes, I've spoken with them," as if she's accepted any outcome.

"I understand his will is still in question?"

"That's true," she says, referring to the marching armies of lawyers and my daughters' war over my estate.

"We'll try not to bother him with too many stressful questions, if he's with us," Eugene says. "Or that's really more advice. There's no telling how he might respond, having been in a coma this long."

"What happens if he doesn't wake up?" Lia asks.

"I think we've discussed that, as well. His medical power of attorney states no CPR, so we'll just see."

"God will decide," she says, authoritatively. Lia always loved doctors but never appreciated anything ambiguous. Which is I guess another reason we were together for so long. Because she never allowed me to half-heartedly love her. And I didn't.

Dr. Eugene doesn't say anything, though her silence does.

"So I guess we hurry up and wait?" Lia punctuates.

"For now, that's all we can do," Eugene agrees.

"If you don't mind leaving me alone with him," Lia continues.

"Of course," Dr. Eugene says. "Let us know if you need anything."

"Thank you, I will."

I feel as though I'm sitting on the other side of an interrogation window now. Except there are no questions being asked of anyone. And Lia is on the opposite side. And somehow we both know the other is there. And we're looking at the window with our hands on the glass. Only one of us can speak to the other. And Lia starts talking.

"Steven," she says. "It's mensch of you to still be here. I know you're in there. Fighting to get back to us. Remember when you fought for me that day in Marin? I knew what was in there that day, too. And I've loved everything, every little corner of your heart, of your mind, and want you to know that I so desperately want you back. Here with us."

It's at this moment I realize that it was that day in Marin that she taught me how to speak. And I tell her by exhaling on my own so that she can tell my breathing isn't controlled by the ventilator.

"Tomorrow we might be a family again for the first time in too long," she continues. "Last week Danny said they're honorably discharging him after the mission he was on. He's going to ask Elie to marry him, and I'm going to allow it. Just think: in a few years we'll be grandparents. I'm going to tell him about that arms company, how they lost their contract. It will be okay, though. We've still got enough. We'll be grandparents . . . Oh, Steve," she clasps my hand within hers. "Please come back to us tomorrow." I feel a tear on my hand, an absolving rain. "Please keep fighting. I've been doing everything I can just to keep it together. You're not alone. I know you haven't been alone. The doctors are doing everything. I've done everything. Steven, please stay alive in there until tomorrow. And come back to us. You're all I've ever had."

She collects herself for a moment. And then she begins to stroke my hand.

"Ferris tells me this Dr. Gideon character wants him to take the thing they're going to use to wake you up global. You're going to change the world, simply by waking up. You're the most high-profile person they've ever used this thing on and the media is going to be here. They're so confident it's going to work that they've invited all the major news outlets. Ferris tells me he'll give us a role, as the spokespeople, ambassadors. Fight for us and fight for this, Steve. I know you can. You've overcome anything you ever set your mind to. Set your mind now to setting your mind," she laughs softly.

But then her tone turns darker.

"If you don't," she says, "then I'll know it's because you can't. I know it's a word you don't have in your vocabulary. Can't. But even the best boat can have impossibly broken parts, like you always said. And if you do, then I'll understand. I'll understand because that's the only possible way I know you won't come back to us. If you can't. But Steve, no matter what happens, know that I've loved you with every fiber of my being, since that day up on that cliff above Marin, since always. Because that day was the first time I saw inside, how beautiful your heart is. Even if you only quoted Jane Austen to impress me," I can tell she's smiling. "And what a life we've lived, together. Forever."

She pauses, as if there's nothing else to say. And there isn't. She just pulls up a chair and takes my hand, stroking it as she used to when she knew my nerves were intruding again. It's something all the money in the world couldn't pay for. The thing that kept me alive all this time. And it's something I'll have again tomorrow. And for whatever life we have left together. Of this I am certain.

THIRTY-NINE

THE BLUR OF ETHAN'S BODY PASSING ME AS I STOOD transfixed served as an awakening. While I still carried a rifle in my right hand, the decision not to take the shot at Ethan or at the bear right away occurred beneath the surface of what I could remain aware of in that moment, where compassion battled greed. My body was reacting to what my brain was doing in a delayed fashion. When I turned to run it felt almost like a reflex. As the bear lumbered on towards us.

Ethan ran limping with his right leg where he'd been clawed the night before. I craned my neck to see the bear escalating its lumbering to a trot that resembled a run.

"Back up the tree!" I shouted at Ethan, about fifteen feet behind him and gaining due to his injury. Somehow, he didn't seem to hear me. "Back up the tree!"

Instead Ethan had turned towards the ravine where snow had piled up, probably six or eight feet deep the night before. Hearing that the bear was now a mere ten or so yards behind us I decided to take cover behind the largest tree trunk I could find, while Ethan continued towards the ravine. The bear chose to chase Ethan rather than me.

I could see everything happening before it actually did. And my mind told me that Ethan was going to die. While he was running the fastest he possibly could, the bear was a mere few yards behind him as he approached the ravine. I readied the rifle again.

But then, and I'm not sure exactly how this happened, how I missed it—my brain must have ignored all other information except that which seemed inevitable—but at that very moment, when I was thinking this to myself, something amazing happened. And that was in the form of a wolf-dog. Nali. That beautiful and wild and more beautiful animal, coming as a blur from the left side of my vision, bearing her fangs and snarling like you've never heard an animal snarl, barreling in a blur towards the bear, distracting it first, and then doing its best to sink her teeth into its front paws, causing the bear to moan and woof and moan some more, to release its own animalistic yawp, and allowing time for Ethan to dive into the ravine, where he disappeared into the collected snowfall, filled in and ten feet deep.

The bear, startled, was initially as shocked as I was, and while I felt an immediate joy at Nali's heroic act, it soon became clear who was probably going to win the battle between the two of them. The bear circled back, its right leg wounded by Nali's tearing at its flesh, and when Nali made another go at the bear, it swung its good paw at her, striking Nali above the left shoulder, and slinging her probably ten feet towards the same ravine Ethan had dived into. At this point I knew if I didn't do something Nali would instead be the bear's victim, and so produced the aught six with my right hand, fully locked and loaded, and fired a shot directly at the bear's hind-quarters, grazing its back not so much that it was incapacitated, rather scaring it as much as it had terrified us. The thousand-pound bear then retreated in shock as I saw Nali crawl towards the ravine, following Ethan, who was silent.

I approached the area of the ravine where Ethan had dived. And there was Nali, lying there like injured animals do, not making a sound because they know they're injured, as she licked the place the bear had gashed her left shoulder.

"Hey, girl," I said. "Oh, look at you."

I then took a few more steps to where I could see the indentations where Ethan had dove. The ravine was deeper than I had thought when I saw it the night before from the tree.

"Ethan!" I shouted. "Ethan?!"

Nothing.

"Ethan!!" I continued to shout, almost frantic. Still nothing. I could see that he'd taken about the first foot of snow off the top of the drift with him before he'd made his way in, and that there was a man-sized area carved out, that descended into what appeared to be a ten-to-twelve-foot-deep chasm.

A million thoughts rushed through my mind—could I conceivably go in after him?—no—could I somehow send Nali after him?—definitely not—what did I possibly have that could extirpate him from the icy death that awaited him?—it was then I had a flash of insight.

We'd brought several ropes with us that were intended as tools to relieve the jeep if it had stuck, things we could tether to the front gate. As the adrenaline began to wear off a little bit, I felt my legs begin to shake, and walking back towards the overturned car I could afford no false or unnecessary movement of any kind.

I reached the destroyed jeep and began mucking around the wreckage, trying to find the ropes. I found the survey films we'd taken were still intact inside the heavy metal box where they'd been kept. It seemed our mission had been accomplished just as the bear had arrived. I thought the ropes had been left in a bag that looked similar to the one our tent came in, and after rifling through all of that size, I still hadn't found them.

By this point Ethan had been in the ravine well over an hour. I turned towards his direction hoping I'd hear something. But still nothing. It occurred to me that the ropes might be buried beneath the jeep, and there might be no way I'd get to them.

Then I realized. Yes, I realized! I'd left them in the compartment in the trunk, beneath the floor board—I remember from two nights ago, after I'd seen the track. I'd made sure they were "safe" just in case we were stranded and had to deal with a bear—instead the bear had been the element of our stranding.

Within a few minutes I was laying on my back in the back part of the cab, my hands thawing enough so that I could manipulate the floor board open, where two twenty-five foot, thick and sturdy ropes fell on my neck and face. I'd never been so overjoyed.

Shadows of what my father had been accused of accompanied me as something deeper towards the center of my consciousness compelled my tying of the ropes as I again reached the ravine.

"Ethan?!" I shouted, less frantic than before.

I looked over at Nali, who appeared worse, as well. Her eyes appeared morose. It occurred to me that no matter what my intentions were, it might not matter. I might just be losing my best friend regardless of what I did or didn't do. The same went for Nali. And myself.

"Ethan?!!" I again let out, more full-throated.

It was then I heard a groan, so soft that I thought it could have just been a limb or a branch in the wind, as it was distant. But unmistakably human. And from a deeper direction, within the ravine.

"Ethan . . . !" I said. And again the groan. "Ethan, I'm going to throw a rope down to you. Grab ahold and I'll pull you out!"

Another groan was followed by a painful gasp, and I knew he'd been injured. I tied the knot as tightly as I possibly could, given my frozen hands; and threw it down into the hole Ethan had carved in the ravine. I had no idea whether he'd heard or understood me.

I pulled the rope back a few yards and felt no tension. The way it was situated I wasn't going to be able to just let it fall back down to him. I reeled it back up, and again threw it down into the chasm. "Grab the rope!" I shouted, hoping that if Ethan was half-awake it might fully rouse him. This time I heard the groan as if responding to my shouting. "Grab it! Put it around you!"

And just like the nibbling of a halibut, deep in an ocean current, this time I felt a slight tension, then stronger, and then a full taking of the object. And I knew Ethan had the rope.

I dug my heels into the foot of snow still on level ground, and heaved with the full force of my legs and back. I'd done this before and it had trained me well to extract my friend from an assured death. The opposite of what it was usually intended for. I heaved again and again, gaining another foot or two each time. I was no longer thinking, purely wrapped in the warmth I felt coarse through my muscles, in perfect unity with my mind and heart. I was determined not to let Ethan die as it rose to the forefront of what I now knew, no longer buried.

By the twelfth heave I saw Ethan's arms holding onto the rope, above where he'd looped it around his back, exactly as I'd told him. With a final effort he slid out of the ravine and onto the forest floor, barely making a sound. Nali had quickened, as well, watching what was happening, and now stood on three legs, the gash burned bright red in her left upper shoulder and flank, no longer bleeding.

"Ethan . . . " I said, rolling him over on his back, where his lips and face appeared blue.

"I'm . . . " he said, attempting to get words out.

"Yes, yes what?" I said, eager.

"So . . . hot . . . " he said.

I remembered that hypothermia, in its final stages, causes people to feel an intense warmth. The sky remained overcast and flurries began falling again, to the left and down, enveloping the forest. Ironically to Ethan's situation and at the core of our collective problem, how to generate heat became a matter of preserving our lives.

I thought that if I drug him back to the jeep first, perhaps getting him inside might save us. And in his condition, I knew that I'd have to be the one to get him there. We had a gas stove that was still working, and I thought I'd seen a hypothermia blanket—the ones that kind of look like foil—there, as well.

"Ethan," I said. "Do you think you can walk? We need to get back to the car."

"I . . . " he said, and then trailed off. It was clear I was going to have to carry him.

"Here," I said, sitting him up. "Get your hands around my neck."

His body felt heavier than it probably did usually, as his muscles were in complete shock. He was able to cling around my neck, as Nali stood and was able to limp along with us.

I scrambled around the wreckage that the bear had left, looking next for the stove and the hypothermia blanket. Nali again lay down, this time next to Ethan.

I rifled through a few bags, finding a pack of smoked salmon in one the bear had opened, but not gotten to. And no blanket. The wreckage was being covered in increasing snowfall and I began to feel desperate. Even if I'd wanted to run some herculean run out of Garland Pass, back five or seven miles in the snow, this was now out of the question, given my recently sprained ankle. I was able to put just enough pressure on it to limp around to the other side, where I found the container for the stove. However, the pipe connecting the gas to the burner had been severed, rendering it useless. There would be no fuel. It was now only the blanket. Which I wasn't even sure existed. It was then I kind of panicked again, anguished, realizing what was probably going to happen to us. Even after coming this far.

The bear had rolled the car away from the forest and towards a clearing, and something instinctively told me to get out there. In retrospect, I wonder if it's because if we were going to die of hypothermia, I at least wanted to have the chance of sunshine when it came back. Maybe thaw us out, raise us from the dead. I tied another end of the rope and lassoed it around myself and Ethan, carrying Nali in my arms, driving like I'd driven the sled during football practice those few years I'd played in high-school. Every ounce of strength leading me into the clearing.

I dragged us to the middle of it, beginning to pray for sunlight, warmth, the only thing that could save us at this point. I'd taken the survey films and stuffed them under my coat, so that they would know we'd succeeded before everything had happened. It seemed equally likely that we would become the bear or another animal's meal before their slumber for the season.

I stopped and produced the smoked salmon from my pocket, tore the packaging with my teeth and ate it like a bear. I took bites in chunks and chewed them, my body having fully returned to where I'd been all those nights ago in San Mateo, after my father had announced I wouldn't take over the company, rendering me impoverished. I thought that if this were my last meal, it'd be a fine one.

I then walked back the twenty or so feet to where Ethan was lying, dying of hypothermia, and set Nali down on him. I pulled his legs up towards his chest and placed his arms crossed in front of him, with Nali on his chest, her fur covering his head. I then lay across his legs and torso, my head on the other side of his back, hunched over and attempting to warm him. I thought if anyone was going to die it should be me, over and over again in my mind, feeling the warmth continue to build as it had. "Let it be me," I said out loud. "Take me. Take me."

Images began to rush in front of my eyes, as my body temperature continued to plummet despite these efforts. I saw Camille and Red and Lia and Kim and Rich Dawson and all the people I'd ever cared about or not cared about, wondering what they were going to think when they heard Steven Levinson and Ethan Helms had frozen to death while surveying for the pipeline. Because they were greedy and ill-prepared. Just as I'd been chasing the salmon that led me here.

I thought about my mother and how she'd been the strongest woman I'd ever known, to leave her homeland, from persecution, to come to a new land and raise me so that I barely noticed what she'd been through, barely noticed what she'd endured, to have endured what my father endured. Though it was my mother's warmth and compassion I felt my mind and heart in those moments.

These hallucinations, as the ones from the plant root in Cao Lanh that never really went away, I knew were based in truth, yet also my growing drift towards unconsciousness. At which point I imagined my suffering would finally end. And in these moments, I began to hear a distant hum. Like the hum of the universe. Not really a hum of any kind, but kind of more a rhythm rooted in the fundamental properties. The way everything is constantly illuminated and humming. Just for existing.

It grew stronger. And then began a kind of glissando effect, up and down, up and down, more quickly, intensifying, up and down, so that I knew the rhythm had two points. An echo. A Doppler. And it continued to grow. Stronger. Stronger. So that I thought it was growing in my brain, the beginnings of unconsciousness. My return soon complete.

And then the wind began to blow, so that it seemed a blizzard was now upon us. Here to bury us. So that we wouldn't be eaten the next day. We were being buried. Nali's head perked up, as the blizzard intensified. Sharp winds began stinging my face in every exposed part. And the hum was now a roar. As I turned to face what Nali was facing, I saw what I had seen so many times in Vietnam. The roar descending from the sky. Those who were supposed to meet us that day, knowing what had come to Garland Pass, had sent a rescue helicopter to extract us from a blinding white death. And I saw for the first time the suffering of the past and present transform in my heart from an eternal void of darkness to an enduring hope.

FORTY

THE FIRST THING I HEAR THE MORNING THEY'RE GOING to wake me up are the reporters with their cameras getting set up in the hallway at Parnassus. It's still early red-black o'clock and they're doing things like white testing their lenses to make sure the reporter's shirts don't appear too visually cloying. There's a rustling within the room, as well, as technicians begin readying the instruments that are going to bring me back. I don't hear a voice I recognize until Dr. Eugene enters.

"We're going to need to pull the tube within the next hour," she says, as if announcing the Israelites will be released from Egypt.

My confidence is at an all-time high.

"That was the plan," Glower says to her, still carrying the air of authority over my care. I suddenly feel where my right fourth and fifth toes are missing, lost to frostbite after what had happened with Ethan. I wondered if Ethan would be present, as I hadn't heard anything. In all honesty other than Lia, Regina, Genevieve, Coraline, Thomas, Elie, and Ferris, and the doctors, I have no idea who'll be here, as Dr. Eugene had alluded to. But I feel an intense joy that the waiting will soon be over.

"Welcome to NBS 7 News," I hear a voice rehearsing in the hallway. I know they aren't broadcasting yet, because they aren't doing anything to me. "We're here outside the Dover Neurological Intensive Care Unit at the University of California-San Francisco Medical Center, to witness a medical miracle that, if all goes according to plan, could rewrite the book on the prognosis of medical coma." It sounds like a beautiful woman. As they all do when you've been incapacitated.

You can hear hushed but growing murmuring both in the room and the hallway as you do when people are getting ready for an event. The kind where you know people are having dozens of little conversations, about strategy, execution, anything that needs to happen to make sure all goes according to plan. And pleasantries. Or as though before a concert performance at the symphony, or the theatre Lia and I used to go to, down the street in Pacific Heights. Season tickets for something like thirty years, to those plays of Beckett and Williams and the bard of Avon, my obsession with the one that brought confusion to Albion. I was obsessed with those moments before the performance, and I'm sensing it now, strangely, anathema to the environment. This isn't a performance of any kind. But I accept it. For the kids who'll know that their loved one can be woken up, too, from this kind of state.

Finally, I hear her voice. "Let's all stand over by the window," Lia says to people I can't really make out through the voices, who must be nurses, techs, other researchers, device company people, and of course the media, who are making a bigger and bigger din in the hallway, preparing to go live. I realize the time must be drawing very near. Hospital administrators, curious kibitzers, I hear them all, their voices making a low murmuring hum, coming to rescue me.

I listen for Genevieve, Regina, and Coraline, but I'm not picking them up. I'm listening for Danny, and I think I just heard him say something to Lia, at which point I think I might wake up right away. No device necessary. But I don't.

"Come over here, Elie," Lia says, and more than only her footsteps approach the direction, towards the window, from which Lia's voice is coming. I feel a rush almost as intense as when I thought I heard Danny at the thought of seeing the unspeakable beauty of The Sunset and Golden Gate Park overlooking the Pacific Ocean. Ocean Beach and The

Cliff House will be one of the first places I go. "Ferris, you too," Lia says through the murmuring. So that I know he's with Elie and Danny.

Suddenly the room grows silent, as it does when everyone's paying attention to something. Like the person who comes out to make announcements before the event. And in a sense this is what's happening, as Dr. Eugene rolls the device into the room. The news units break into a full-throated broadcast at what's about to occur.

"In just a matter of moments," the woman's voice says, now in the room, as I feel the cameras for the first time, their steady heat, "Mr. Steven Levinson, Chief Executive Officer of the Noble-Dyer conglomerate, a ten-billion-dollar enterprise, including oil and natural gas, wineries, fisheries, as well as ownership of information and biomedical research technologies, will be subjected to a revolutionary new technique, called ultrasonic thalamic stimulation. Mr. Levinson has been in a coma after an accident in the Queen Charlotte Islands for the past six weeks. His wife, Lia, daughter of the famous neuroscientist, Karl Goldberg, has asked for the media to be present, so that the world might become aware of this new technology. With potential to rewrite the book on prognosis for patients in Mr. Levinson's condition. I'm joined by Dr. Jane Eugene, pioneer of ultrasonic thalamic stimulation here at UCSF. Dr. Eugene, can you explain what's about to happen?"

"Sure," she says. "And thank you for being here. We wouldn't normally do something like this, though Lia insisted that this is what Steve would have wanted. And we're all excited to share the potential of ultrasonic thalamic stimulation with the country, and indeed the world.

"Basically, we're going to introduce sound waves to a place deep in Steve's brain, called the thalamus, which is a center deeply rooted in consciousness. As has been demonstrated in clinical trials and the device recently approved by the FDA, patients in Steve's state should regain theirs with use of this device."

"Amazing," the beautiful voice says. "Is there anything else you'd want the public to know before we get started?"

"Just that," Dr. Eugene says, "—as you'll see, when Steve comes to, that this could be your loved one someday. Don't give up hope. Never give up hope."

"Okay," the voice says. "Well, we'll leave it up to you, after a brief commercial break."

The cameras' light-heat dissipates for a moment.

"All right," Dr. Eugene says, "—let's extubate."

And like the first rain in a desert after six years of drought, I feel my nemesis begin to slide out of my breathing passages, the tissue feeling like its being born again. The intense newness of the ambient atmosphere tingles tenderly for a mere moment, before it starts to itch not from irritation but from sensitivity. As the tube slides out of my mouth and I feel my tongue unimpeded for the first time in six weeks, the first thing I do is cough a little.

"That's encouraging," Glower says. "It means his lungs are strong."

"How much time before we should come back on the air," the beautiful voice says.

"Just a minute or two. Let's make sure he doesn't lose the contents of his stomach," Glower says.

"Okay," she says.

And so here I am. Six weeks removed from Thomas's and my shipwreck, breathing on my own again. No tube. No machine. And I already begin to feel the resemblance of humanness again. Like I'm not a cyborg. Or a mere object to which things are done.

"I think we're ready," Eugene says.

"All right," the voice says. "Maybe it's a better shot if he's already wearing the device when we return?"

"Okay," Eugene returns.

And then I feel the device being lowered onto my head, with a kind of rubber-Styrofoam padding that feels pretty pleasant.

"We'll need to position the stimulators," Eugene says. And for a few seconds she's adjusting the padding. "Based on our measurements from the last MRI, this should be the angle."

Silence for several moments.

"All right," she says. "I think we're ready."

The voice cues the heat again, as the red-black is almost completely red. For some reason flashes of what I imagine I'll see won't come to my mind as they had before, as at the outset when I could basically imagine anything. I'm also not seeing shapes. Just intensely red red-black. For a split second I feel intense fear. But then a pleasant calming as the heat warms my newly shaven face. My shorn hair.

"Dr. Eugene, we're ready when you are," the voice says with the cameras rolling.

"Okay, ladies and gentlemen," Dr. Eugene says. "We're going to wake Steve up now. Should only take a minute."

I hear the click of a switch, and then the low humming like the helicopter, except I know this time it's a different kind of wave coming from above. I feel the vibration of the device through the rubber-Styrofoam intensifying, a car reaching speed.

And then it begins. Like a black and white film becoming in-color—no, like a painting or relief emerging from a canvas—no, like peering through bushes and then removing them with your arm, to reveal what was a blind man's view of a canyon's panoramic depth, and all happening faster than a child's blinking eye, I have regained my vision.

As I begin to track the room, seeing faces and colors brighter than ever before, a round of applause circulates as well as several gasps and other sounds of awe. I try to say something. I'm not there yet. While my hearing has always been acute, it is now even more so, as I hear a monitor from three doors down remind me of what I'm leaving.

In front of me are Lia, Elie, Ferris and his father, Danny in uniform, Thomas, as well as my team of doctors.

"Steve," Dr. Glower says. "Steve, you're back!"

I again try to say something but can only moan.

"It should take a minute for him to be able to speak," Eugene says.

In that moment I can't really explain what it's like, only that I feel like a little baby. Like my eyes are consuming everything, reorienting everything, putting things back together. I'm amazed when someone out of the corner of my eye drops their pen and notepad. I see Ken and Ed and Ted out of the other corner of my eye, and Lia smiling at me, her little baby. I raise my right arm like I want to put it in my mouth, but stop myself, then feeling a little older. Maybe a toddler. I want to get up and run and run and run, throw things, and I have thousands and thousands of questions.

My first question is why Dr. Glower's eyes have been restored, but I can't ask it. I want to know where Genevieve, Regina, and Coraline are. I want to know why Thomas is here and not hiding as Ferris said he would be. Oh, I have so many questions!

"Steve?" Lia says. "Steve, I love you. Can you say you love me? Love us?"

"I . . . " my first word emerges, "—love . . . "

Another round of gasps and applause circulate. The camera's lights are blinding. "Ladies and gentlemen, Steven Levinson is awake," the voice of the woman who is as beautiful as I'd imagined, auburn hair on her dark olive complexion.

"Where—" I draw a breath, practicing speaking, "—where . . . "

Yes, Steve, you're in the hospital at UCSF—" though all I want to know are where Genevieve, Regina, and Coraline are.

"Where are our daughters?" I manage to say, as Thomas looks at Elie, who looks at Ferris, who looks at Danny, who does not look back at Ferris. Danny looks at me in full fatigues with a concerned expression, but doesn't say anything. I fixate on him until Lia speaks again.

"Our daughters?" Lia says.

"Where are our daughters?" I repeat.

"Steve," Lia says, confused. "Is he okay?" she asks Dr. Eugene, who's again standing next to Dr. Glower, whose eyes appear completely normal.

"Steve, what daughters are you referring to? Maybe he means something else," Dr. Glower says.

"Genevieve, Regina, Coraline," I say. "Where—" I continue, really wanting to know.

"Steve, we don't have any daughters," Lia says, looking confused. "Just one son, Danny," without acknowledging him.

I see Dr. Eugene motion to the cameras to stop filming.

"And so you have it," the beautiful reporter says kind of nervously, as though she's done something wrong. "A medical miracle! Amazing! Stay tuned to NBS News 7 for further coverage of Steve's evolving condition. We'll be back again with an update tonight, at 7."

The heat of the cameras goes away, as the hum of the device and my disorientation continue.

"Our daughters," I say again, with more force, my lungs remembering how to speak.

"Steve," Lia repeats, "—Steve we only have one son, Danny," she looks at Eugene again.

"But they all want control of the company," I say. "They thought I would die."

"Steve," Lia says with more emotion, "Steve. For the last time, we don't have any children other than Danny." And I look again for Danny, but this time he's not there. Only Ferris, Elie, and Thomas.

"Then where—Dr. Glower?" I say. "And his children—Ed and Ted?"

"This is Dr. Darren Anders," she points at Glower. "This is Dr. Jane Eugene. Dr. Anders has a son, Henry, who was your medical student," she points at Ted who said "Poor Tom". "And this is your nurse from St. Mary's, Martin." She points at Ed.

"But—" and I can't muster the strength to clarify anymore.

"Danny is on his way to see you," Lia says. "He's going to be here this morning."

"Oh," I say, letting go a little of my need to see our daughters.

Lia looks at Eugene again, as if something's not right.

"Why does he think we have daughters? Who is Dr. Glower?" Lia says.

"It's normal for people's brains, when they're in comas, to make up for what senses are lost," Dr. Eugene says. "I've seen this before."

Dr. Anders comes over to me, this time with caring force. "Steve," he says. "Steve I've been with you since day one, over at St. Mary's. You're in the Dover ICU at UCSF. Your only child, Danny, is on his way to see you. You don't have any other children."

"He was always obsessed with a Shakespeare play," Lia says. "The one with the old king. That must be what he's referring to. He thought he was the old king before this happened."

Eugene nods knowingly as Lia's phone rings.

"Here," Lia says. "See? It's Danny!" As I try to understand why Danny was just next to Ferris. "I'll step out for a minute."

"Steve," Dr. Eugene says. "You're now an international miracle."

"That's great," I say, trying to be genuine.

Suddenly I see that Danny has reappeared next to Ferris, again looking at me with concerned eyes. As though he knows something I don't. Lia enters again after a minute or two. I can see the tears well up her eyes.

"Steve," she says, her voice cracking, "—Steve, something terrible has happened."

I feel my heart race for several beats, then return to its normal rhythm.

"Steve," she says, looking at Elie and Ferris and Thomas, transfixed,"—Steve, Danny's been killed," and her emotion bursts through. "That was the Colonel," she says. "He was killed in a raid outside Kabul three days ago." I turn and see Danny standing next to Ferris, for the first time noticing a red spot on the upper left portion of his uniform.

"No," I say. "No, he's here," again with more force, looking directly at Danny.

"He's hallucinating again," Lia says through tears. "Just like he thought we had daughters."

I see Dr. Eugene cringe and frown, as if this is what she didn't want to happen when they woke me up. Something stressful. I'm now not gazing, not looking, but staring at Danny. The expression on her face is unchanged.

"So now we have no children," I say, still staring.

Lia can't say anything. She's crying, so intensely that the heaves are coming from her stomach. She's happy to have me awake, but overcome by the devastation at Danny's having become a casualty of the war in Afghanistan. Our only son.

I again feel my heart racing for a few more beats, before returning to normal. I'm short a few breaths before they pick back up again. The pure joy I felt at returning is now another shipwreck, a turbulent sea, pulling me to shore.

Elie joins Lia in her bursting emotion, Thomas joins them, all hugging next to me. I see Ferris grin. I feel my own emotion, now more mature, as if I'm thirty years old. I'm getting older. Closer to my age.

My heart races for twice as long as before. My breath is again, short. I know what I need to do. Tears stream down my face, and I cough, knowing that if I let it take ahold of me fully, it'll come sooner. My only son is dead. My heart continues to race, weakly.

"Lia," I say, as my tears halt momentarily. "Keep as much as you need to live a wonderful life . . . Give half of what's left over . . . to a woman named . . . Kira Bugaev . . . She was born in . . . Fairbanks . . . around nineteen seventy . . . Her mother's name is Natalya . . . Tell Kira to give . . . half to her mother and uncle, Vladimir . . . Give the other half to . . . Thomas Mariner."

Lia approaches me. "Can we take this off?" She asks.

Dr. Eugene approaches and does what she says. She says how sorry she is for what's happening to her with her facial expressions. Danny is gone, and I know he'll remain gone until it's time.

"Steve," she says, sensing my shallow breathing. "Steve, the money's almost gone, too. Remember, you sold your share when you said production had been cut by half since the eighties, and you put your money into that arms company supplying the war. They lost their Pentagon contract this spring. Remember?" My heart is now continuously racing, as shallow as my breathing. My skin, which had felt like I'd just showered, now feels like it's going numb again. And I know it's coming, creeping from my toes to my knees and legs, from my hands to my elbows and shoulders, leaving only my neck and my head. Creeping piece by piece.

I remember now, in my aged madness, before I sent Danny, or convinced Danny to send himself, to suffer as I had, Lia was right—I had gotten out of Alaskan oil and into arms to supply the fight in the Middle East. And knew, before I drowned to enter what had been that play's apparition, I might end up financially where I'd begun. The remainder of the businesses were almost completely borrowed against on credit, including the one in the Islands. Which I'd wanted to give Thomas, to hide it from Danny. In wanting to support the war he was fighting in, I'd needed to hide from him.

"Steve—" she says smiling through tears, "—Steve: go."

I take one breath as deeply as I can. Feeling Danny's death and the loss of my fortune at once.

"Lia," I say with only enough for a few more words. "I'm sorry . . ." I feel the air burn my heavy lungs, "You saved me… Now . . . save yourself . . ." And drawing what I know will be my last, "I'll . . . love you forever."

And with that I feel myself let go. Not intentionally, but taking in the full weight of what I'd endured. What monitors are left announce it. I rise out of my body, suspended, an apprehending eye, free from matter.

What they say about your life before you die is true. I saw it all, from the trees outside our house in Anchorage, playing with Ethan as a small child, how my eyes were mere moments ago, the look on my mother's face when I learned to ride a bike, the tadpoles I caught from the pond, the girls in elementary school calling me names, how my mind had returned to where it came from after Stanford, my first rebirth in Vietnam with Camille Le, the first breath I took in San Francisco when the war was over, everything passed before my eyes, watching Danny learn to play baseball, ride his own bike, try to make me proud.

And then as I remained there, sensing Danny's presence but not seeing him, in my hospital room at Parnassus, truths began to fall, washing over my soul like rain. I had left Danny out because I'd been left out. I'd sent him to war because I'd been sent to war. I wondered if he'd forgive me. For not knowing until now. That my father had left me out because he was trying to protect me from what he'd done. That making it in the world the way I had was better than the alternative. I wondered if Camille would forgive me for thinking I could save her—that we could save each other. I wondered if the play Lia and I had seen a thousand times about the old king, and that my brain thought I needed at St. Mary's and up until now had truly prepared me. What vanity and insanity I was protecting.

And then Danny was there again, standing next to Thomas at the foot of my hospital bed. Motioning for me to come with him. Showing me where I would go. Where we would go.

I was standing with Lia on the cliff in Marin after our first kiss, the Pacific Ocean a panoramic scene so beautiful and glistening as to defy words. Danny was with us then, as he had arrived when my spirit left my body, greeting me, waiting for me, showing me where to go. And we were on the cliff above Marin. Redolent breeze and birds, seagulls and pelicans passing by. Riding waves of wind. Danny nodded. And we jumped.

We fell with speed and force, knowing that we could not die because our bodies were dead already. Mere matter from which we'd found freedom. We fell into the San Andreas fault, falling deeper and faster, plunging through crust and layers, first arriving at the center of the Earth, at its core, which was spinning hot and lava-golden. We remained there for a moment, then passing through an opening in space that was taking us still deeper, through a portal that dug farther and farther, directing us towards the center of the universe, where I understood we would encounter the center of consciousness. Together.

We flew with force from the Earth and through space, towards the center, so that star dust was left in a trail, first at the speed of light and then slightly slower, so that we could still see each other's spirits in the corporeal world. Danny was illuminated and calm and peaceful, and he looked over at me, smiling. For the first time since the accident, I smiled. We were warm in the vacuum of space. We were headed towards the center.

As we made our approach an object appeared in the cosmic distance, only just visible. It was a black hole with the mass of several galaxies, of eighty-six billion stars. A disc of light was circling around it, with all frequencies of the invisible spectrum now visible. Colors were each complete in prisms, with a central intense beam radiating from the center of this gargantuan object of undulating space. I had reached the center of consciousness.

Flying still faster and somehow suspended, now in communion with the center, I first became aware of numbers, first zero then one and one and two and three and five and eight, I could process everything with numbers, including the harmonies of the stars as they sang through space. I then became aware of every color, every sound, I heard each sound and saw every sight I'd ever seen and heard, felt the tactile warmth of the stardust all around me, tasted each flavor from bitter to sweet, felt and saw and heard and tasted. I tried to process with numbers these senses and then understood not to, to let processing power and my senses remain independent but united forces. I processed not only with what I saw and heard and tasted and felt. But I also sensed still deeper, a layer beneath, emerging from these senses, anger and sadness and joy and laughter and surprise and love and compassion, and rolling combinations of each. They were each their own form of feeling, their own primary color, while remaining also independent of the numbers and processing. I did not judge which were good or bad, only knowing that they were and that I was, both receiving and giving these qualities to the universe.

As the black hole grew closer and we approached its event horizon, the point of no return, I became fearful and suddenly my mind became mute—and then out of the silence I finally found words. Not words of themselves, but more like the shapes that make the forms of words—at the center were words. Space where there was a lacking. To be filled with a word. Beautiful and ugly and biting and ultimate, all forms were words, even symbolic and musical forms. All had language.

With Danny I had arrived at the center of my consciousness, seeing the black hole at the center of the universe. There we were arrested for a cosmic year, and I felt that at my core, whereas I had reason when on Earth to doubt, was care and compassion, it had been turned from anger and fear, and always unbridled ecstasy at the lifeblood I'd been given. At the opportunity to live. It was this I'd given Danny. The black hole I understood now was massive but not black. And I hoped that this was where we'd remain for all eternity. I saw Danny glowing golden next to me. Enraptured by something only describable as a sense too deep for words, that I'd only felt for him and Lia. And I knew then it was the reason I had been on Earth.

But our journey was not yet complete. While Danny had been there, waiting for me in my hospital room after his death, there was a place I must go alone. Led by him and leading him, where we'd go together, separately, before a hopeful reunion. Rather than descending into the center of consciousness, into the black hole at the center of the universe, as momentum directed us towards the event horizon, rather than be strung out and sucked in like a piece of thread, we instead were diverted to an elliptical ricochet, a whip of an orbit so powerful and fast that it took less than a millisecond, at which point our spirits were slung around and destined for the outer reaches of space.

The force of our spirits' slinging was such that we crossed in front of each other, to one side and then the other, star dust paths trailing and the heat generated by the discovery of what was at the core of our hearts radiating waves warming planets, passing nebulae birthing stars, nebulae like animals with octopus arms and crab's eyes, neutron stars spinning and quasars emanating, brilliant towering plumes of life-stuff and stellar matter obeying the laws God had set for them. I understood these were the same objects I had imagined the first time Lia allowed me to kiss her, and seeing them with Danny was like a homecoming.

I knew that I was responsible to these objects. To the awe of stars and moons and planets and comets, just like Danny and me, to the love I had felt for Lia and would always, the only eternal thing, the generating force which had brought Danny's spirit to Earth.

I passed galaxy after galaxy, past the point of Earth and our nearest neighbors, faster than the speed of light. And only after this, I lost Danny in my spirit's vision. I was only aware of him but could no longer see him, like in waning dusk light, somewhere he was off in the woods while eighty-six billion stars shined, blinding me. I was reaching my destination. Where everyone has to go eventually. Alone.

After I had seen all there was to see, heard and tasted the primordial tastes, knew the universe and myself, felt the eternity of love and compassion, and ceased caring what came next, it was then that I realized I was approaching the outer limits of space. It was calm and peaceful, as I found hope and pity and honor and sacrifice resided there. The summation of eighty-six billion stars, connected. At the outer limits I found them, shimmering in flux, showing me what it was to be human. And in my own perseverance in the face of cosmic fate, cosmic struggle, I found victory only in perseverance until death, final forgiveness, before all began falling away—all senses and calculations and actions and words and meanings and all time, that emergent property of matter—piece by piece, as my body had before.

And my spirit was then peaceful, resting alone in a room, vacant but for a chair and a window air conditioner in the desert, blowing softly on my sweat-drenched neck, a naked lamp in a corner illuminating itself and the room. Long vacant shadows were cast of the chair I was sitting in, but I had no shadow. I was alone in this room in the outermost sky. I stood up and approached an open wall, my spirit now horizontal with the now absent floor, seeing only intense stars.

I grew closer and my soul was still, and still closer to the open wall, realizing I had approached the outer limits and was close enough to almost reach the expanding edge with my out-stretched arm. And I began to ask: what it is expanding into? Into what is the universe expanding? I knew only that this was where I was going. Where all souls go. Where all questions will be answered. And when answered they will cease to haunt. And it grew silent but for the roar of my mind about to depart.

Danny had waited for me, and as the force grew still stronger on my head, now crushing magnetically, I hoped that if I made it through to the other side I could wait for others. I wondered if Camille Le and my mother would be waiting for me. I wondered what my father would have to say when he finally met Danny. If he would forgive us for never knowing his haunting, a foreigner come to a strange land.

The sound escalated, beginning as a dull roaring. I had only time for a few remaining thoughts. I understood the play, the core of my obsession, had prepared me to forgive them and myself—as all the ones I'd seen had in some way, and the ones that lived on would continue to for generations and generations. Before I had blamed everyone and then myself. It had prepared me in this moment and then forever to blame no one. As I left the open room, approaching the outer limits, my hand now inches away, I blamed no one. Which is the only way one can pass through, I realized.

I then saw the outer limit of space, expanding barely in front of my eyes. The sound grew deafening, a siren reaching peak intensity. It was dark, and beyond there was what it was and had always been expanding into. Some believe it is empty, but I sensed, had faith before that final instant that it was full. The place into which I would be passing was full. There was no beginning and would be no end. I looked back behind me and saw the light of the universe receding to a single point, the naked light of that room illuminating itself and the universe. From the black hole in the center to the edge which I could feel with my hand. Almost touching what it was expanding into.

The sound roared. I closed my eyes as my soul crossed the outer limits in silence in a flash of light separating two eternities.

ACKNOWLEDGEMENTS

It takes a village to create a book. Thank you to the members of the village who made *Stage of Fools* possible, beginning with Scott Wolven and Shanna McNair for their faith in my writing over the years, and for sharing their vision, expertise, and community with me and so many others.

The idea for this book sprang forth from conversations with Rick Moody on the nature of consciousness, after a workshop during the pandemic; can't thank you enough, Rick, for lending your generosity and genius; hopefully we've proven that dark times can bring forth bright things.

Thank you, Stephen Jan Parker, my academic mentor, for teaching me to both believe that a dual career in literature and medicine was possible, and for imparting that porous Nabokovian worldview which unites the arts and sciences; other indispensable mentors without whom this novel would have been possible include David Bergeron, who taught me how to read Shakespeare and write a good sentence, Katie Conrad, James Carothers, Mary Klayder, Dr. Howard Nash, Dr. Jeff Burns, Dr. Terrie Mendelson and the whole UCSF-St. Mary's academic team, as well as Drs. Paisith Piriyawat, Salvador Cruz-Flores, Gustavo Rodriguez, Anantha Vellipuram, David Briones, and the whole Red Raider neurosciences community.

This book delves into the emerging issue of Neurorights and the evolving definition of what it means to be human; specifically, the issue of mental augmentation. Heartfelt thanks to the Neurorights Foundation, including Dr. Rafael Yuste, the Santiago Ramon y Cajal of our time, Jared Genser, and Jamie Daves for your faith that we could get the law passed in Colorado last year; to Senator Cathy Kipp and Governor Polis; and to Lukasz Szoszkiewicz and Stephen Damianos for your unwavering leadership and support. May the trilogy raise awareness, encourage the adoption of, and add to the narrative of the greatest technological advancement and human rights issue of our time.

None of this would be possible without my friends and family—first and foremost my wife, muse, and emotional rock, Jen; thank you for your undying support, courage, and inspiration, for making sure we live well, persevere, and return to the Italian countryside. Thank you to to Mom, Peter, and Dana, and to my friends who've been there throughout the journey: to PJ Barnett, Chris Pavlacka, Grant Randall, Rebecca Evanhoe, Grant Schoenebeck, Matt Davis, Matt Pirotte, Sean Murray, Jon Carnell, Jordan Chance, Korak Sarkar, Alex Geng for your insight, and to Mark Michalski. Thank you Bruce Plankington, Roger Fincher, and the crew for the unforgettable adventures to the Queen Charlotte Islands, at the base of Alaska.

And finally to Dad, who encouraged me to write since that first novella in middle school—to seek adventure, and to dream.

ABOUT THE AUTHOR

Sean Pauzauskie was born in Anchorage, Alaska, and raised in Topeka, Kansas. He was educated in Kansas, California, and Texas, and holds an honors degree in literature. He was mentored by and wrote his thesis with Stephen Jan Parker—a favorite pupil of Vladimir Nabokov—who encouraged him to "get a day job" before writing seriously. He became a practicing neurologist as a result of this advice. Including *Stage of Fools*, he has written five novels, a collection of short stories, an autobiography and a work of drama. He lives with his wife and Siberian husky in the foothills of the Rocky Mountains, where he enjoys fishing, sports, traveling, composing piano music and mountaineering. His literary scholarship has been presented in such places as at the International Vladimir Nabokov Society Conference in Montreux, Switzerland. Learn more at seanpauzauskie.com.

Stage of Fools is his debut novel.

www.ingramcontent.com/pod-product-compliance
Lightning Source LLC
Chambersburg PA
CBHW020501310726
48979CB00016B/2750/J
* 9 7 8 1 9 6 2 9 3 1 3 1 1 *